ASSESSMENT OF HEARING DISABILITY

Guidelines for medicolegal practice

Inter-Society Working Group on Hearing Disability

Air Vice-Marshal P. F. King, CB, FRCS (Chairman)
King Edward VII Hospital
Midhurst
West Sussex GU29 0BL

R.R.A. Coles, MB, FRCP(Ed)
MRC Institute of Hearing Research
University Park
Nottingham NG7 2RD
(representing British Association of Otolaryngologists)

M. E. Lutman, PhD (Secretary)
MRC Institute of Hearing Research
General Hospital
Nottingham NG1 6HA
(representing British Society of Audiology and British Association of Audiological Scientists)

Professor D. W. Robinson, DSc, CEng
Audiology and Human Effects Group
Institute of Sound and Vibration Research
University of Southampton
Southampton SO9 5NH
(representing British Society of Audiology)

Professor R. Hinchcliffe, MD, FRCP
Formerly: Institute of Laryngology and Otology
330/332 Gray's Inn Road
London WC1X 8EE
(representing British Association of Audiological Physicians
until his retirement in 1991)

ASSESSMENT OF HEARING DISABILITY

Guidelines for medicolegal practice

P. F. King, R. R. A. Coles, M. E. Lutman and D. W. Robinson

Whurr Publishers
London

First published 1992 by
Whurr Publishers Ltd
19b Compton Terrace
London N1 2UN, England
Reprinted 1993

British Library Cataloguing in Publication Data

A catalogue record for this book is available from the British Library

ISBN 1-870332-04-0

Printed in the UK by Athenaeum Press Ltd, Newcastle upon Tyne

Preface

This book came into being following decisions by the governing bodies of those professional associations most closely concerned with the medical and scientific assessment of hearing loss, and its effect on the individual. The Inter-Society Working Group on Hearing Disability, which was formed from the nominees of the four relevant Societies or Associations, has met on 25 occasions, and over a period of 5 years the work has taken shape. From the start it was decided that any recommendations should be based on known scientific data. This has necessitated a major search through the literature, and the comparison and assessment of data available. This revealed inadequacies in the then current literature, which led the Working Group to undertake new scientific work. As a result, several original or review papers have been published or accepted for publication.

Although it was the original intention to prepare a report, with recommendations, for submission to each of the four professional associations, it became evident with the passage of time and the development of ideas that much new ground was being broken. Because of this, it was believed that the work would have much more validity if it was published under the names of the members of the Working Group* as its authors, rather than as an anonymous report. Although the original sponsors have requested the report, what follows in the completed work is the responsibility of its authors. We hope that it will be endorsed by the professional associations.

There are also practical reasons for the authors assuming responsibility for the work. No-one would claim perfection in any task undertaken by humankind, but what is presented to the reader is the result of much work and considerable discussion. Circulation of the Report for comment and arriving at a consensus before publication would surely have led to delay, and might cast what has been done into desuetude.

It should be emphasized that the Report is the joint work of the authors, though different members, singly or together, have had the task of drafting different chapters: it has been our aim to write a composite account, and this is not a collection of individual papers.

It is hoped that the readers and users of this work will be helped by its contents. Doubtless, time and practice will indicate faults and errors, but these should not detract from the main thrust of the recommendations which are made.

P. F. King
Chairman

* In addition to the authors, Professor R. Hinchcliffe was a member of the Working Group, representing the British Association of Audiological Physicians, until his retirement in 1991. During his period of membership he contributed much useful advice and constructive criticism.

Preface

Contents

Chapter 1 Introduction

1.1 Historical background and terms of reference

In 1981, a member of the British Association of Otolaryngologists (BAOL) wrote to the Council of the BAOL pointing out the multiplicity of, and conflict between, the various published recommendations on assessment of hearing disability for compensation purposes. He asked BAOL if it could give some authoritative guidance on this. A working party was set up to consider the matter and the British Society of Audiology (BSA) was invited to participate and nominate one or two representatives. The resulting working party (P.F.King and R.R.A.Coles from BAOL, and W.Burns from BSA) published its report, commonly referred to as the 'Blue Book' (Anon, 1983). It was well received by some, but with misgivings as to its content, rationale or representativeness by others.

Accordingly, in 1985, with new research data available from D.W. Robinson and colleagues at the Institute of Sound and Vibration Research of the University of Southampton, and from the Medical Research Council Institute of Hearing Research in its multi-centre epidemiological studies, the Council of BAOL decided to initiate the setting up of a further working party to examine the new evidence with a view to reconsidering the joint BAOL/BSA recommendations. In doing so, it decided it would be helpful to widen the representativeness of the working party and accordingly invited the British Association of Audiological Physicians (BAAP) and the British Association of Audiological Scientists (BAAS) to participate and each to nominate a representative. After discussion between these various organizations Air Vice-Marshal P.F. King, CB, OBE was asked to chair the new working group.

The first meeting of the working group was held on 25 June 1986. That meeting agreed the following:

(i) That a detailed review was desirable and timely.
(ii) That the working group would be called the Inter-Society Working Group on Hearing Disability
(iii) That its terms of reference would be:

> To establish the need for and to propose a method for the quantification of hearing disability resulting from hearing impairment for the purposes of description and compensation, with particular reference to noise-induced hearing deficit, and to report.

These terms of reference were subsequently accepted by the parent organizations.

The Inter-Society Working Group on Hearing Disability held 25 meetings in the period 1986 to 1991, in the course of which a thorough examination was made of the many aspects of the quantification of hearing disability. The material that follows comprises the report and recommendations of the Working Group.

1.2 Scope of Report

This Report proposes a method for the quantification of hearing disability* resulting from hearing impairment* for the purposes of description and compensation, with particular reference to noise-induced hearing deficit. The scientific and technical background to assessment of hearing disability is reviewed. Methods of measurement of hearing impairment for the purposes of medicolegal disability assessment are defined and guidance is given regarding problems associated with such measurements. Means of allowing for coexisting impairments, primarily due to ageing and conductive hearing loss, are described. Formulae and tabulations are given for converting measures of impairment into estimates of percentage disability. Rules for apportioning disability between two or more exposures to damaging noise are described and the issue of prognosis of future disability is addressed. Various worked examples are given in Appendix A. Recommendations are summarized at the end of the chapter in which they occur, and also at the end of the Report.

1.3 Rationale and philosophy

Ideally, hearing disability assessment should provide an accurate quantitative assessment of the actual disability experienced by the individual, appropriately weighted according to the way he uses his auditory faculties and the extent to which difficulties in hearing interfere with those activities. This is unattainable by strict scientific method and the proposals described in this Report deliberately do not attempt to tailor disability assessments to individuals: individuals vary widely. The report focuses on the typical (median) person† and attempts to provide an assessment which would apply to that notional individual. The consequence of this is that assessments will carry an element of 'rough justice'; a person who is genuinely more disabled than would typically occur for a given hearing impairment will be assessed too conservatively, whereas a person who is genuinely less disabled than would typically occur will be assessed too generously. This has been accepted because, at the present time, there exists no method of measuring disability directly in the individual which is face-valid, acceptably accurate and adequately representative.

The decision to focus on the median person was mainly a consequence of three fundamental decisions at the root of this Report. The first of those decisions was to base the recommendations primarily on scientific data: much of previous recommendations has been based on opinions, even though these were from experts in the relevant fields. We were able to do this principally because a large amount of data concerning hearing impairment and hearing disability has become available from the

* These terms are used with special meanings defined in Chapter 2.

† In this context 'median person' refers to one whose reponses on the various measures specified in the Report correspond to the 50th percentiles of the distributions of these measures in the (notional) population of persons having similar descriptions and history.

National Study of Hearing conducted by the Medical Research Council Institute of Hearing Research during the early 1980s. The second decision was to base assessment of hearing disability on measurement of hearing impairment (see definitions in Chapter 2), given the relative precision and verifiability of the latter. Thus, a relationship between disability and impairment was required based on measurements in order to convert impairment measures (pure-tone hearing threshold levels) into disability estimates. Because of the large element of measurement uncertainty inherent in most general measures of disability, it was necessary to extract the central tendency from rather large groups of subjects to arrive at reliable estimates of disability for the typical individual; this entailed concentrating on median data rather than on other percentiles of the distributions of scores, which tend to combine true dispersion with measurement uncertainty. The third decision was to use self-reports of disability, rather than disability measured in terms of performance on certain specific auditory tasks, such as speech identification in noise. The former has the major advantage for our purposes of face-validity, but has a disadvantage in terms of greater measurement uncertainty. This reinforced the need to concentrate only on median values.

A further advantage of self-reported disability for our purposes was that we were able to use a set of quantitative self-ratings of hearing in which large numbers of subjects had rated their hearing ability on a scale from 100, meaning normal for a young person, to 0, meaning totally deaf. This lends itself naturally to a disability scale measured in percentage terms, which was a principal requirement of the assessment scheme.

When the assessment scheme is used to quantify the disability arising out of a certain cause, such as exposure to noise or injury to the ears, the concept of the median person is invoked in another way. In general it is not possible to know what the hearing status of the individual would have been if the cause of the hearing impairment had not occurred. This is particularly so for gradual impairments such as those arising out of occupational noise exposure over long periods. Hence the individual being assessed must be compared with a notional individual of the same age and sex, but without the cause of hearing impairment. This requires baseline data for subjects representative of the general population, but without the cause of hearing impairment in question. Usually this amounts to a database for subjects with no known cause of hearing impairment other than normal ageing. Once again, there is an element of 'rough justice'. The individual being assessed may have had particularly good hearing before exposure to the cause of impairment and, although the status of his hearing without exposure is unknowable, it might be expected to have been better than the median. By the same argument, an individual who had poor hearing before exposure or who was more than averagely susceptible to the ageing process might be expected to have worse hearing than the median person even if he had not been exposed. For these reasons, it is possible that a person who is genuinely damaged by exposure to a particular cause of hearing impairment may still retain better hearing than the median person of the same age and sex and thus be deemed to have no resultant disability. For complementary reasons, it is also possible for a person who sustains only slight damage due to exposure to be deemed to have a substantial resultant disability. These limitations, which are common to most assessment schemes, should be borne in mind when dealing with individuals. They have been deliberately accepted in order to achieve a relatively simple and workable system of assessment. The recommendations can only deal with the general case: exceptional cases must be argued on their own merits.

The final major element in the rationale of the assessment scheme is that differences between the (exposed) individual being assessed and the notional (non-exposed) median person are computed in the domain of disability rather than impairment. Thus, in order to calculate the attributable disability, first the measured impairment of the individual concerned is converted to a disability estimate. A corresponding conversion is then made for a notional person, or 'control'. The control has the median hearing impairment expected in a person of the same age and sex, plus any additional components of hearing impairment from non-attributable causes that have been measured in the individual concerned. The *attributable* disability of the individual is the difference between these two estimates.

Summary of chapter recommendations

- Assessment should focus on the disability expected in the typical (median) person for a given degree of impairment.
- Indirect assessment of disability via a (verifiable) audiometric surrogate is necessary in the absence of any satisfactory method of direct assessment.
- Allowance for age-associated hearing loss should correspond to the impairment expected in the typical (median) person of the same age and sex (notional control subject) as the claimant.
- In making such allowance, by comparing the claimant with the notional control subject, differences should be computed in the domain of disability.

Chapter 2
Definitions particular to this report

Terms used in this Report are mostly based on general usage or definitions by authorities such as the World Health Organization (WHO), British Standards Institution (BSI), International Electrotechnical Commission (IEC) or International Organization for Standardization (ISO). The Glossary towards the end of the book contains various terms used. However, in preparing the Report, it was found to be necessary to coin certain new terms, or to expand, restrict or qualify existing definitions. The following definitions are particular to this Report.

air–bone gap
For the purposes of this Report, an air–bone gap is taken to be the average over the frequencies of 1, 2 and 3 kHz and applies to measurements obtained using the methods of audiometry specified in this Report. (See also Glossary.)

apportionment
In this Report, apportionment is deemed to be in the disability domain. (See also the Glossary.)

attributable hearing disability
The hearing disability attributed to the alleged injury or disease and to any other injury or disease of like nature; for example, attributed to two or more periods of noise exposure or between two or more separate head injuries.

binaural faculty loss
The loss of the advantages conferred by binaural hearing, the advantages being equivalent to improvements in signal-to-noise ratio, and which deteriorate with increasing asymmetry of hearing. One component arises out of the head shadow effect; another arises out of the binaural squelch effect sometimes referred to as the 'cocktail party effect'.

binaural sensitivity loss
A loss of sensitivity for free-field sounds under binaural listening conditions which increases with increasing asymmetry of hearing. In the extreme case of asymmetry occurring when one ear is normal and the other is totally deaf, binaural listening is the same as monaural listening. The difference in loudness between binaural and

monaural listening conditions for a person with two normal ears is equivalent to approximately 10 dB.

constitutional hearing disability*
Hearing disability arising out of constitutional hearing impairment (see below).

constitutional hearing impairment
Hearing impairment due to disease, degeneration or other process that is not connected with the alleged injury or disease leading to the claim for compensation, or any similar injury or disease. This will usually comprise age-associated hearing loss and any conductive hearing loss present, but for the purposes of this Report it could also include other incidental forms of injury: an example is a total unilateral hearing loss due to previous head injury which would be discounted in a case of alleged noise-induced hearing loss in the other ear.

genuine hearing threshold level
A hearing threshold level that is not spurious (see below).

hearing disability
Restriction or lack, resulting from a hearing impairment, of ability to perceive everyday sounds in the manner that is considered normal for healthy young people.

hearing handicap
A disadvantage for a given individual, resulting from a hearing impairment or hearing disability, that limits or prevents the fulfilment of a role that is normal (depending on age, sex and social or cultural factors) for that individual. Being a psychosocial concept, it is not capable of direct measurement and cannot be inferred completely from the disability assessment. For the purposes of this Report, therefore, measures of hearing disability are used in preference to measures of handicap.

hearing impairment
Abnormality of function of the hearing system. There are many forms of hearing impairment that could be measured; these lie in the intensity, time and frequency domains and include non-linearities. The relationships of many of these to disability are largely unknown and none has been shown to be superior to pure-tone sensitivity for estimating disability. Therefore, for the purposes of this Report, hearing impairment is quantified solely in terms of pure-tone hearing threshold levels.

noise-induced hearing disability
Hearing disability arising out of a noise-induced hearing loss. For the purposes of this Report, noise-induced disability is defined as the difference in disability estimated from the overall hearing thresholds of the noise-exposed individual and the disability estimated from the thresholds expected in the median person of the same age and sex not exposed to noise together with any other constitutional hearing impairment. Negative noise-induced disabilities are deemed to be zero.

---

* These definitions apply only for the purposes of this Report. The same terms are used with a different meaning elsewhere.

prognosis*

Prediction of disability generally, or at a specified time, usually under the assumption that there will be no further cause of hearing impairment other than normal ageing. The prediction depends on a model of how pre-existing impairment and age-associated hearing loss summate. There has been no generally accepted model up to the present time.

spurious hearing threshold level

A hearing threshold, measured or reported, that does not reflect the intrinsic sensitivity of the ear in question. It is usually in the direction of a greater apparent hearing loss than the genuine hearing threshold level.

* These definitions apply only for the purposes of this Report. The same terms are used with a different meaning elsewhere.

Chapter 3
Technical background

3.1 General

In order to fulfil the aims of this study, a thorough examination was made of the scientific basis for quantitative disability assessment. A substantial amount of relevant new material came to hand during the lifetime of the Working Group, and where such material has been relied upon in formulating the present recommendations brief particulars are given at the appropriate places in the text. Some aspects entailed decisions based on reviews of past work. A summary of the matters considered by the Working Group is given in the following sections.

3.2 Surrogate measures of disability

A key decision which influenced much of the detailed work was to give preference to the self-rating of disability as the basis on which to erect a quantitative scheme, whilst recognizing that this method is not an appropriate instrument for direct application to individual cases, particularly in the context of claims for compensation. In practice, this meant the selection of an appropriate surrogate measure and the establishment of a population norm for the relation between self-rated disability and the surrogate. As in virtually all previous schemes, the choice of a surrogate came down finally to one or other index derivable from the pure-tone audiogram. Other measures were considered, including various psychoacoustic tests of cochlear function, but were not found to be sufficiently well-founded or to give a better representation of hearing disability.

3.3 Characterization of the concept of hearing disability

From the earliest days, the assessment of hearing disability has conventionally been identified with loss of speech perception and given quantitative significance by performance at a speech test. Average performances of test groups were compared with their average audiometric impairment to derive an indirect scale of disability. This view of what constitutes disability is deeply engrained and runs as a common thread from the pioneering work of Fletcher (1929) through six decades. It has formed the basis of innumerable schemes, differing only in the conditions (implied or explicit) in which the speech performance is measured and in the extent to which the results of scientific experiments have been simplified to provide administratively attractive formulae. This last step marks a distinction between disability and what might be termed 'deemed disability' for purposes of administering a compensation scheme, a point to which we return in 3.6.

Details of the genesis and metamorphosis of these disability scales have been given, among others, by Suter (1978) and by Hardick et al. (1980). These accounts serve to demonstrate that no consensus can be arrived at as to which is best from all perspectives; for example, applicability to different types of hearing loss or at different levels of impairment, or for compensation as opposed to hearing loss prevention.

The attraction of an integrated measure of disability, obtained by some form of self-assessment, is that it avoids prejudging which, out of an unlimited variety of speech perception tests, in quiet or in various types of background noise, should be taken as representative; indeed, it avoids the question of whether speech perception is the main or sole basis on which people judge their hearing ability (even leaving aside individual psychological reactions which fall in the domain of 'handicap').

To sidestep reliance on average relations between disability and audiometric impairment, questionnaires have been devised from time to time intended for direct application to individuals, an example of these being the hearing measurement scale (HMS) described by Atherley and Noble (1971) and Noble (1978). Whatever the merits of such instruments for correctly rank-ordering people's degrees of hearing disability, they cannot form a rational basis for quantitative evaluation because the methods of scoring responses and summing over questions are necessarily arbitrary. Moreover, such questionnaires are open to abuse in the medicolegal context. Furthermore, it has repeatedly been observed that correlation between questionnaire-based self-report and speech–hearing performance is no better than, indeed usually inferior to, that between self-report and an appropriate audiometric impairment measure (Coles, 1975; Noble, 1978; Tyler and Smith, 1983; Robinson et al., 1984; Lutman et al., 1987). According to Coles, 'it could be that the measured impairment [the reference here being to HTLs averaged over 1, 2 and 3 kHz] is in fact a better guide .... than the patient's description of his hardship'.

Given that the practical implementation of a disability assessment scheme necessarily reduces to the employment of an audiometric surrogate, these results clearly point to a further potential advantage of self-report over speech performance tests as the basis for establishing the norm for a disability scale. The objection to questionnaires, that they are non-metrical, is dispelled if the self-assessment is itself made in quantitative terms. This device combines the merits of face validity with the direct delivery of a quantitative scale. The method was successfully employed by Habib and Hinchcliffe (1978), using two sample populations of clinical subjects. A similar technique has subsequently been used on a large sample representative of the general adult population (Lutman and Robinson, 1992), and the results from that study have been adopted for this Report.

3.4 Audiometric descriptors

A wide variety of audiometric descriptors has been advocated at different times and places for best representing performance at speech tests, usually taking the form of simple averages of HTLs at frequencies within the range 0.5–6 kHz, but sometimes with weighting factors or other refinements. Despite 60 years of endeavour, no final agreement has emerged as to which is the best descriptor.

The historical accounts of the various proposals, given in the references mentioned above, reveal certain trends but also a number of internal contradictions regarding the optimal combination of frequencies. Among the complications there is the finding that the 'centre of gravity' of the frequency range used in the descriptor tends to move towards lower frequencies as HTL increases (Webster, 1964). However, the details of these indices, their relative merits in different circumstances and conditions of speech testing, and the minutiae of their comparisons with one another, become largely irrelevant when the basis of disability rating is broadened by the adoption of self-assessment. It is pertinent, therefore, to examine experimental data from those studies which have employed self-assessment and which also provide comparisons between different audiometric descriptors. Four such studies are considered below.

(a) Atherley and Noble (1971) applied the HMS to 38 persons suffering from NIHL. Five out of the seven sections of their questionnaire are relevant to disability, viz. 'speech hearing' (both quiet and noisy situations being represented); 'acuity' (hearing for non-speech sounds); 'localization'; 'speech distortion' (referring to the quality of the speech); and 'personal opinion'. Correlation coefficients between scores on these categories and various audiometric descriptors are given in Table 3.1 (columns headed SH, A, L, SD and PO, respectively).

(b) Lutman et al. (1987) derived four principal components from the responses of 1470 people to a questionnaire. Three of these components are relevant to disability, viz. 'everyday speech', 'speech in quiet' and 'localization'. Correlation coefficients are given in Table 3.1, in columns ES, SQ and L, respectively.

(c) W. I. Acton (personal communication, 1986) calculated correlation coefficients for the results of 120 subjects suffering from NIHL, with disability ratings based on the self-assessment questionnaire described by Kell et al. (1971). These results are given in Table 3.1 in column A/K.

(d) Included in the National Study of Hearing was a question for the self-rating of hearing ability of the participants on a scale of 0–100. The correlation coefficients between these ratings and various audiometric averages for the better ears of 2058 subjects were calculated for the purposes of this Report, and are given in Table 3.1 in column SR.

The results shown in the table clearly indicate the high importance of 2 kHz. Acton's correlation coefficients differ only marginally among themselves and, although the differences may not be statistically significant, they suggest that the correlation is diluted by the addition of lower frequencies to a greater extent than is made up for by averaging over adjacent frequencies (compare (a) with (g)). Those combinations containing 4 kHz are slightly less favourable than those with 3 kHz (compare (d) with (c)

Table 3.1 Correlation coefficients relating self-assessed disability and various audiometric descriptors.

	Frequencies	Atherley and Noble					Lutman et al.			Acton	NSH*
	(kHz)	SH	A	L	SD	PO	ES	SQ	L	A/K	SR
a	2(alone)									0.66	0.63
b	0.5,1,2	0.51	0.64	0.63	0.19	0.19	0.63	0.39	0.35	0.58	0.65
c	0.5,1,2,3	0.49	0.58	0.53	0.58	0.49				0.62	0.66
d	0.5,1,2,4						0.62	0.39	0.33	0.60	0.66
e	0.5,1,2,3,4	0.40	0.53	0.69	0.59	0.48				0.63	
f	0.5,1,2,3,4,6	0.40	0.51	0.46	0.62	0.54				0.64	0.65
g	1,2,3						0.59	0.37	0.31	0.64	0.66
h	1,2,4						0.60	0.36	0.31	0.62	0.65
i	3,4,6	0.28	0.34	0.41	0.55	0.38					0.60

* Data from the National Study of Hearing (M. E. Lutman, private communication, 1991).

and (h) with (g)). The whole-audiogram average, (f), shows no advantage over the combination 1, 2, 3 kHz (g), which again suggests that any advantage in averaging over more frequencies is offset by including those at both ends of the range. Atherley and Noble's results for the 'sensitivity' categories, SH and A, appear to confirm the impression that adding extra frequencies does not improve correlation: note the descending values in (b), (c), (e) and (f). The converse holds for SD and (almost) for PO, whilst the results for L show no progressive pattern. The data of Lutman et al. show only small variations with frequency combination, but a slight preference for combination (b). Those authors caution that differences of 0.03 between correlation coefficients in the region of 0.6 are only on the borderline of statistical significance. From the ensemble of data, the balance would be slightly tilted in favour of (b) according to Lutman et al. and part of Atherley and Noble's HMS findings, but towards the inclusion of a higher frequency on the basis of Acton's results and, more particularly, the SD and PO categories from the HMS where the combination (b) showed up very poorly. The results from the numerical self-rating question in the National Study of Hearing, on the other hand, vary so little with the frequency combination (with the possible exception of the 3, 4, 6 kHz value) as to suggest that the choice of frequencies is indeed largely arbitrary.

The evidence reviewed is clearly insufficient on its own to compel a decision on the frequency combination, but there are other considerations to take into account. These arise from the fact that the disability scheme has to be used for assessing individual cases, by inferring a notional disability from a set of actual measured HTLs. The first of these considerations is that 0.5 kHz is among the less reliable frequencies as judged by repeatability trials, second only to 6 kHz in this regard (Robinson, 1991a). Secondly, in the case of NIHL there is often a notch in the audiogram, usually in the vicinity of 4 kHz. These notches are sometimes narrow in the frequency dimension but may be quite deep (20 dB or more). There is, therefore, a chance of obtaining an inflated HTL measurement which does not properly characterize the average level of the audiogram in the region of the notch. This is much more likely to happen with the 4 kHz audiometric frequency than with 3 kHz. Another incidental advantage, but one which is quite important in practice, is the relative difficulty of measuring accurate bone-conduction thresholds above 3 kHz (Coles et al., 1991).

These practical matters, in conjunction with weak indications of a strictly scientific nature, led the Working Group to adopt the three-frequency average, 1, 2 and 3 kHz. This should not be construed, however, as implying the absence of *any* disability in some individuals with hearing losses restricted to frequencies outside this range.

An incidental advantage of this selection is that it accords with UK practice in statutory hearing loss compensation and standards for hearing conservation, and thus may lead to easier acceptance than has attended departures from established practice in the past. There are examples of such changes being made on very dubious grounds, for example when CHABA (1975) responded to a request to change the hitherto widely accepted AAOO recommendation (0.5, 1, 2 kHz) by substituting 3 kHz for 0.5 kHz in such a way as to result in the same compensation costs; the report of the CHABA working group offers no convincing reason for the change but they nevertheless acceded to the request. In the UK, the predecessor to the present Working Group recommended in their draft report the continued use of the 1, 2, 3 kHz combination, but this was overturned by the sponsoring bodies. These dissenting voices may have been influenced by the then recent work of Suter (1978) whose correlations for a group of mildly impaired persons pointed in the direction of 1, 2, 4 kHz. The limited scope of Suter's tests, however, led Hardick et al. (1980) to remark that her 'conclusions may not be generalizable to individuals with more severe hearing losses affecting the low frequencies'; their own preference was for the five-frequency average, 0.5, 1, 2, 3, 4 kHz with a fall-back recommendation of 1, 2, 3 kHz if, as they suspected, the inclusion of 4 kHz would give rise to (non-scientific) objections. These remarks are given simply as a commentary on the slightness of evidence that has swayed previous groups charged with reviewing the problem of disability assessment, not as corroborative evidence for the particular combination chosen here, because data on self-rating did not feature in previous reviews.

3.5 Scale relationship between audiometric impairment and disability

Quasi-quantitative unidimensional measures of disability derived from summing the responses to multi-item questionnaires, as in the HMS, provide a scale with ordinal (rank-ordering) properties only; there is no way of knowing the cognitive distances between the scale points. Scales derived from percentage-correct scores at specific speech tests are less arbitrary, but no scale of this kind is unique because the test conditions radically affect the scores obtained. Consideration was therefore focused on direct quantitative estimation of disability, by the only means available; that is, by numerical self-rating of perceived disability. Habib and Hinchcliffe (1978) applied this method to two clinical populations, one in London and one in Cairo. The impairment was represented solely by the HTL at 2 kHz and the correlation with subjective magnitude was 0.315 ($P<0.01$). Results for the two populations were similar in form but differed by a factor of about 1.5 on the subjective magnitude scale, the London contingent yielding the lower ratings. The method of analysis used by those authors was constrained to represent the relationship between percentage disability and HTL as a progressively accelerating function, and thus was unsuitable for extrapolation in the higher ranges of HTL. The National Study of Hearing provided data on similar lines for a much larger and more representative population sample, and the results have been analysed by Lutman and Robinson (1992), using a mathematical model better adapted to accommodating results over a wide range of HTL, using the 1, 2, 3 kHz average HTL. The resulting function is given in Chapter 8.

3.6 The low fence and the high fence

There is a wealth of experimental evidence pointing to there being a continuous variation of disability with increasing HTL, whether the disability is measured by self-rating or by some form of performance test. Despite this, much effort has been expended on defining two points on the HTL continuum, below the first of which ('low fence') disability is deemed to be absent and above the second of which ('high fence') disability is deemed to be total. Three distinct ways of specifying the low fence are outlined below

(a) An impairment-based low fence is that value of HTL at which hearing is significantly different from normal. Normal here refers to the zero reference level as specified for audiometers together with the statistical distribution of HTLs for young, otologically unimpaired persons. Significantly different from normal means lying beyond a specified, but arbitrary, fractile of this distribution on the positive side of zero, for example the 90th, 95th or 98th percentile. The cut-off point is a matter of judgement, and has never been uniquely specified.

(b) A performance-based low fence is arrived at by choosing a fractile of the distribution of scores at a test (such as speech audiometry) given by young, otologically unimpaired persons, and then translating this value back to HTL using a pre-established median relationship between HTL and score. This definition was adopted by Robinson et al. (1984); it has the attraction that the low fence so arrived at is much less dependent on the nature or difficulty of the speech test than the actual error scores themselves. It leads to considerably higher values for the low fence than by definition (a) for the same selected percentile.

(c) A disability-based low fence can be defined in the manner of the study by Merluzzi and Hinchcliffe (1973), using subjects' responses to a dichotomous question on the lines 'Is your hearing normal or not?'. Normalized distributions of the HTLs of those answering yes and no respectively intersect at a value of HTL which becomes, by definition, the low fence separating the able from the disabled in a statistical sense. This method appears to yield lower values than either definition (a) or definition (b)

It can be seen that, whichever definition is taken, the process of arriving at a low fence is highly arbitrary, which raises the question of whether it is necessary or desirable to postulate this concept at all in the context of hearing disability assessment. The same applies to a high fence.

The literature is quite clear on this point: the fences are erected as an administrative convenience. They have been introduced at the expense of fidelity to the true nature of things, either to satisfy a demand for simplicity or (at the low end) to get away from trifling monetary awards and vexatious claims from individuals with hearing bordering on the normal. The high fence has often been set at rather low levels as a way of making up for the exclusion of other cases below the low fence. Davis (1971) described a well-known two-fence scheme in these words: 'In the interests of simplicity, the AAOO rule introduced unreal abrupt transitions at zero and at 100% handicap [disability in current terminology]. From the point of view of the victim, the rule is harsh at the low fence but lenient at the high fence.' High fences have ranged from as low as 70 dB HL (average at 0.5, 1, 2 kHz) upwards. It is obvious that hearing impairment is not total at that level, and consequently that disability is not total either. At the low end, fences as high as 50 dB HL (average at 1, 2, 3 kHz) are to be found (e.g. in the UK statutory compensation scheme, although 50 dB is the point of entry and relates to 20% disablement). Even at the lower value of 26 dB (average at 0.5, 1, 2 kHz) – the value that prevailed for many years in the AAOO scheme – there is no doubt that many persons in this condition are not 100% able in their hearing, especially those who began life with hearing equal to or better than the reference 'normal' for whom a low fence of 26 dB represents a large erosion of their 'hearing reserve'.

There are, nevertheless, circumstances in which the defining of a low fence is appropriate. This is the case, for example, in the control of industrial hearing loss where minor degrees of impairment, and hence slight disabilities for the most susceptible individuals, are an economic inevitability. It is therefore useful to postulate a cut-off point and to work backwards from this to the noise exposure limits that should not be exceeded. Such arguments, however, apply in a broad-brush manner to noise-exposed populations: they have no place in the assessment of the disability of individuals.

In regard to individual assessment, and its sequel in setting quanta of awards, it is important to keep in mind the distinction between 'disability' and 'deemed disability' referred to in 3.3. It should be emphasized that this Report is principally concerned with the latter, in that the individual measurements of hearing threshold level which are made are used to infer a value of disability from a knowledge of the average relationship between the two. This Report is not the place to make specific recommendations about the estimation of disability taking unquantifiable personal factors into account.

It is pertinent to point out here the implications of the system proposed in this Report, which admits neither a low nor a high fence, but only a curve of disability against HTL which starts from the lowest point on the acute side of the young normal distribution (–10 dB HTL) and rises continuously. On the face of it, this scheme would appear to attribute a finite percentage disability to any claimant still within the 'normal' range. However, the disability for compensation purposes is, in fact, to be calculated as the difference between the value on the curve and that for the notional average person, unimpaired except for AAHL, of corresponding age and sex to that of the claimant.

3.7 Differential weighting of the two ears

There is a long history of procedures designed to allow for inequality of the two ears. Fletcher (1953) recognized that two distinct factors come into play compared with the case of ears of equal sensitivity. The first of these, binaural sensitivity loss, is illustrated by the following. Total monauralization entails a loss of loudness, which can be determined by monaural/binaural loudness comparison experiments; it follows that partial loss in one ear can then be represented by a correspondingly smaller loudness loss. Inseparable from this effect is the second factor, binaural faculty loss, manifested as a diminution, or even total loss, of the faculties inherently dependent on the possession of two ears, namely localization and the capacity to resolve spatially separated competing sound sources. Fletcher's solution to allowing for the binaural faculty loss was simply to double the loudness loss, but this was a conjecture without any experimental foundation.

Fowler (1942) devised an empirical scheme based on three premises:

(a) the difference between 'better' and 'worse' ear becomes progressively less important as the better-ear hearing loss increases;

(b) with one normal ear and the other with no hearing at all, the disability is worth 10%;

(c) with one ear totally deaf, the growth of disability increases with the loss in the functioning ear in a sigmoid fashion, the growth rate being greatest between 30 and 50 dB.

This system appears to have originated from a mixture of intuition and clinical experience. Sabine (1942) introduced a more complex variant of Fowler's method while conceding that there was next-to-no experimental basis for it. These systems did not find favour with the American Medical Association (Bunch et al., 1942) who simplified it to a simple 7:1 weighting of the disabilities for each ear, in favour of the better ear; this weighting is apparently still current in the State of Oregon.

Subsequent history is mainly a variation upon the AMA method, with different values for the ratio. In 1959, the AAOO proposed 5:1, which was accepted by the AMA, and has remained in force. Other values have been used, for example 4:1 (Ginnold, 1979), and 1:1 (Hardick et al., 1980). The last-mentioned argued for 1:1 on the grounds that it avoided the 'trap opened by the extreme case of the total unilateral. Weighting the ears differentially to produce a binaural percentage loss that looks reasonable in terms of handicap [disability] for unilateral cases implies acceptance of equal handicap [disability] for equal percentages no matter what the audiometric configuration. We simply do not know enough about differential weighting or how it should vary as a function of severity of the loss to satisfactorily resolve the problem in any but the extreme case'. It is true that experimental data are scanty, but to shy away from the problem in the above manner is not satisfactory in view of the manifest inequity of an equal-weighting rule.

In the UK, the ratio 4:1 was adopted in 1973 in connection with the then DHSS statutory compensation scheme for occupational deafness, but it did not appear explicitly in the regulations until 1983 (Statutory Instrument 1094, at schedule 2A part III).

There is a report (P.C.Robinson, 1978) of an attempt to resolve the binaural weighting problem experimentally, using a questionnaire applied to a sample of 282 subjects, which was said to show that 'the better ear was four times as important in day-to-day functioning as the worse ear'. Reference to the paper cited (Macrae and Brigden, 1973), however, fails to throw any light on how this conclusion was arrived at.

The present authors considered that Fletcher's original proposal, described above, had a more rational basis except for the arbitrary way in which he had been obliged to allow for the binaural faculty loss component. Since Fletcher's time, a certain amount of experimental data has been published on this aspect (MacKeith and Coles, 1971). Accordingly, for the purposes of the present Report, a synthesis has been made of these data with Fowler's premise (a) referred to above plus a component of loudness loss on the lines given by Fletcher. The resulting system is described in 8.3 and incorporated into the tables of disability.

3.8 Age-associated hearing loss

In contrast to the topics already discussed, age-associated hearing loss (AAHL) is a well-researched field, but there are considerable variations between the results of the several dozen systematic studies reported in the literature. Much of this variability can be traced to differing criteria of subject selection, and ethnic differences also appear to play a part. Fortunately, the search for representative results is greatly facilitated by reference to two sources which sum up the state of the art up to 1987; during the lifetime of the present Working Group, a further large body of data came to hand from the National Study of Hearing. A brief summary of these three data sources is given below. A feature common to all of them is a distinction between the AAHL in males and females.

(a) International Standard ISO 7029:1984 and its technically identical counterpart BS 6951:1988 give values of AAHL as deviations relative to the median thresholds of young otologically normal subjects (that is, very nearly but not exactly 0 dB HL). The values refer specifically to screened populations, described as 'otologically normal' except, of course, for the age-related loss. The precise meaning of this can only be inferred from the descriptions of the test populations given in the original papers on which the Standard is founded. Not all of these descriptions are as explicit as might be desired, but at least some degree of subject selection had been made in every case to exclude factors such as known adverse otological history, regular noisy employment etc. The analysis of the original data was described by Robinson and Sutton (1978, 1979).

Values of AAHL are defined for the age range 20–70 years, for percentiles of population from the 5th to the 95th (of which only the 50th – the median – concerns us here), and for audiometric frequencies from 0.125 to 8 kHz. The Standard gives the generating equations as functions of age and percentile, for each sex, and the same data have been published as a set of complete tables for ready reference (Shipton, 1979).

(b) Conscious that the 'otologically normal' population of ISO 7029 was, by design, not representative of the population as a whole, a set of results corresponding to (a) was evolved by Robinson (1988b) for a 'typical population'. Obviously that is a looser concept than 'otologically normal' and liable to be more dependent on the particular population selected for study. In practice, the available results for the largest population samples (some 80 000 people) were of American origin. In the paper cited, these data were analysed on the all-ears basis, that is, two values per person, and as in ISO 7029, these results were expressed as threshold deviations from median normal hearing at age 20. Corrections are also given for conversion to standard HTLs; these corrections are quite small except at 6 kHz where they are about 5 dB; for the average at 1, 2 and 3 kHz the corrections are only 0.2 and 0.3 dB for the male and female populations respectively; these corrections have been applied in column (b) of Table 3.2. The values cover the age range 20–70, percentiles from the 5th to the 95th, and audiometric frequencies from 0.5 to 6 kHz.

(c) The National Study of Hearing obtained data on over 2000 subjects randomly selected from the population of four cities in the UK. The data provided profiles on various anamnestic and audiological variables such as noise exposure history, material conductive hearing loss, socioeconomic status, to mention but three, in addition to pure-tone audiometry. It was therefore possible to select subpopulations by specifying relevant criteria and to examine the distributions of HTL in each. For the purposes of the present study two such selections were made: (i) the total sample for which audiograms were available for both ears, and (ii) the sample remaining after exclusion of significant reported noise exposure and presence of material conductive hearing loss (defined by an air–bone gap exceeding 15 dB averaged over 0.5, 1 and 2 kHz). For both samples, subjects were first sorted according to sex and decade of age and their HTLs were then averaged over 1, 2 and 3 kHz. Distributions of these averaged HTLs were then determined in each subsample. In the case of sample (i), three such distributions were calculated, namely those of the 'better' ears (n=2678), of the thresholds averaged over left and right ears, and of all ears (n=5356) (A. C. Davis, 1988, personal communication). In the case of sample (ii), only the distribution for 'better' ears (n=1746) was calculated because it had become clear that this was the more appropriate specification for a 'reference population' in connection with disability assessment.

A comparison of the three data sources is given in Table 3.2. Columns (b) and (c) (all ears of typical populations) are in very good agreement taking into account the completely independent sources of these data (see column (h)), particularly for the males. Comparing columns (d) and (c), the selection of the better ears leads to lower median thresholds by about 1.5–3.5 dB, the difference increasing with age as might be expected. The elimination of conductive losses etc. further reduced the median threshold for males, but not for females (compare columns (d) and (e)). Finally, comparing the NSH 'better ear' selected sample (column (e)) with the international standard value for otologically normal persons (column (f)), good agreement is again found for males and a rather surprising constant difference of 3 dB for females. For the purposes of this Report, it was considered that the standardized values given in ISO 7029 form the more appropriate baseline for use in connection with disability assessment in individual cases.

Table 3.2 Comparative data on median age-associated hearing loss expressed as hearing threshold levels (dB).

Age (years)	Typical population (Robinson, 1988a)	NSH* (total sample) All ears	NSH* (total sample) 'Better ears'	NSH selected sample 'better ears'	Otologically normal population (ISO 7029)	(e) minus (f)	(c) minus (b)
a	b	c	d	e	f	g	h
Males							
25	3.6	4.4	2.9	1.9	0.2	1.7	0.8
35	5.9	6.7	5.0	4.2	2.0	2.2	0.8
45	9.9	10.9	8.6	6.5	5.3	1.2	1.0
55	16.3	16.7	13.8	10.4	10.1	0.3	0.4
65	26.1	24.1	20.7	17.4	16.4	1.0	−2.0
Females							
25	2.5	4.7	3.0	3.3	0.0	3.3	2.2
35	4.2	6.4	4.9	4.7	1.4	3.3	2.2
45	6.4	8.7	6.8	6.8	4.0	2.8	2.3
55	10.1	12.7	10.0	10.2	7.7	2.5	2.6
65	16.5	19.3	16.1	15.7	12.6	3.1	2.8

* NSH = National Study of Hearing.

Summary of chapter recommendations

- Preference is given to data on the self-rating of disability in the determination of the relation between disability and impairment, as opposed to measures based on performance tests.
- The preferred audiometric surrogate for disability is the average of the pure-tone thresholds at the frequencies 1, 2 and 3 kHz.
- The scale relationship between disability and hearing threshold level that should be used is curvilinear over the whole range and derived from experimental data.
- A concrete proposal is made concerning disability when the sensitivity of the ears is unequal. This involves adjustment for the loss of binaural sensitivity and also the loss of suprathreshold binaural faculties which assist in localization and processing signals in noise. (The adjustment for loss of binaural sensitivity is given by Equation 8.3. This, and also adjustment for loss of supra-threshold binaural faculties, is embodied in Table A2 of Annex A.)
- Allowance for age-associated hearing loss should be according to ISO 7029.

Chapter 4
Audiometric equipment

The procedure described in this Report is based on the pure-tone hearing threshold levels at three frequencies, 1, 2 and 3 kHz. Air-conduction values will be required in all cases. With few exceptions, bone-conduction values will also be required. The requirements below are therefore based on the assumption that both measurements are frequently (even routinely) to be made. This particularly affects the standard of quiet required: the testing room should be regarded as an essential part of the equipment (see 4.6). Some indications are included for additional equipment, useful for diagnosis; in case cortical evoked response audiometry (CERA) is employed, the required standard of quiet is the same as that for pure-tone audiometry (see 4.3).

4.1 Equipment for air-conduction audiometry

The air-conduction audiometer should conform with the specification for Type 1 or Type 2 audiometers given in BS 5966.

> Note 1: audiometers marked with the obsolete frequency series including 1024, 2048, 2896 Hz etc. should not be employed. These older instruments may not comply with current standards in other respects.

The earphones should be of a type providing a direct link to the standards of audiometric zero (see 4.4). The types in most frequent use are the Telephonics Corporation TDH-39 and TDH-49 with the soft rubber cushion type MX-41/AR. Note that the type of earphone determines the type of calibration equipment required to verify the acoustical performance of the audiometer. The use of noise-excluding earphone enclosures is not recommended, due to the uncertainties of fitting and difficulty in calibration. The background noise requirement should be met without the aid of such devices, few of which are effective in any case.

> Note 2: current production of the TDH series earphones is fitted with a new-style cushion, type P/N 510 CO 17 (also known as Model 51); this has been deemed acoustically equivalent to the type MX-41/AR.

The earphones should be fitted to a headband which is adjusted to provide the correct force of application to the subject's ears (4–5 N).

4.2 Equipment for bone-conduction audiometry

The bone-conduction audiometer should conform to the specification for Type 1 or Type 2 audiometers given in BS 5966. Desirably it should be the same instrument as used for the air-conduction testing in order to minimize systematic uncertainties arising from the tolerances which are permitted on individual instruments (see 5.2.1). Narrow-band masking noise having the characteristics specified in BS 7113 is required. The bone vibrator should be of a type with a plane circular driving area in conformity with BS 6950, and fitted to a headband providing the correct force of application to the subject's mastoid prominence (nominal value 5.4 N). Hearing-aid type vibrators are unsuitable; they do not comply with the standard.

Note 1: the recommended vibrator is the type B-71 manufactured by the Radioear Corporation. The type B-72 also complies with the standard but is heavier and more difficult to fit properly; its greater dynamic range at low frequencies is not required for present purposes.

Note 2: the earphone used for delivering the masking noise to the non-test ear may be of the insert or supra-aural type (see 4.4).

4.3 Additional equipment

The following items of equipment may be useful as diagnostic aids.

Sweep-frequency audiometer. This type of instrument should comply with BS 5966 and provide both continuous and pulsed tones.

Note 1: instruments of this type may not lend themselves to the standard practice of calibration.

Note 2: with the exception of instruments provided with narrow-band masking noise that tracks the stimulus tone, sweep-frequency audiometers are not appropriate for testing where contralateral masking is required (as in the determination of bone-conduction thresholds of individual ears) because the correct ('plateau-seeking') masking levels cannot be implemented in synchronism with the continually changing frequency of the test tone (see 5.1.2).

Speech audiometer. Instruments of this type should comply with the requirements of IEC 645-2 (in draft) or its subsequent BS counterpart.

Aural acoustic impedance/admittance instrument. Instruments for measuring the acoustic characteristics (impedance, admittance, equivalent air volume etc.) of the middle ear, and for testing the acoustic reflex, should comply with IEC 1027. Publication of a corresponding British Standard is expected.

Apparatus for electric response audiometry (CERA, ABR etc.) There are at present no standards for such equipment, but a specification for the relevant test stimuli is at the international draft stage. In the meantime, pure-tone stimuli for CERA should comply with the relevant clauses of BS 5966.

Apparatus for tinnitus assessment. No standards exist for equipment of this type. If a pure-tone audiometer is employed, it should comply with BS 5966.

4.4 Coupling devices required for calibration of audiometers

Air conduction. For audiometers equipped with American earphones of type TDH-39 with appropriate cushions (see Note 2 of 4.1) or type DT-48 (German) earphones, calibration is effected using an acoustic coupler complying with BS 4668; for other types of earphone or earphone/cushion combinations, an artificial ear complying with BS 4669 has to be used.

Note 1: verification of the sensitivity of the microphone of the coupler or artificial ear and its associated amplifiers requires the use of a pistonphone or sound calibrator complying with BS 7189.

Bone conduction. Calibration of bone-conduction audiometers is effected using a mechanical coupler complying with IEC 373:1990 (2nd edition) which is identical to the corresponding British Standard, BS 4009:1991.

Note 2: the mechanical coupler specified in BS 4009:1991 differs in important respects from that specified in the previous (1975) edition of the standard, which has been withdrawn. Instruments complying with the new standard are available commercially.

4.5 Quality assurance

4.5.1 General requirements

It is essential that the medical examiner liaises with the appropriate department or individual to ensure that the proper quality assurance applies to each and every test. Quality assurance in this context includes calibration of the relevant equipment and operating methods for the equipment in accordance with the relevant standards, codes and guidelines appertaining at the time.

4.5.2 Principles of calibration

Air conduction. The standard reference zero for the scale of hearing level is specified in BS 2497 Parts 5 and 6 (according to the type of earphone). These standards give the sound pressure levels produced in the acoustic coupler or artificial ear respectively, by earphones of the appropriate patterns, when excited electrically at a level corresponding to the hearing threshold of young otologically normal persons.

Note 1: the acoustic coupler and artificial ear are not interchangeable. The standards specify different sound pressure levels, but these correspond to the same median threshold levels in human ears.

Bone conduction. The standard reference zero is specified in BS 6950, in an analogous manner to that for air conduction in BS 2497. The standard gives the vibratory force levels, expressed in decibels relative to 1 μN, transmitted to the mechanical coupler, when the vibrator is excited electrically at a level corresponding to the hearing threshold of young otologically normal persons. The values given in the standard refer to the vibrator being applied to the mastoid prominence with a static force of 5.4 N and the non-test ear being masked by narrow-band noise at a level of 35 dB above the pure-tone threshold of that ear at the frequency concerned. The specified vibratory force levels apply to bone vibrators having a plane circular driving face with an area between 150 and 200 mm^2.

Note 2: the masking noise level used to define the audiometric zero above is for reference purposes; it will not necessarily correspond to the level required to obtain the true bone-conduction hearing threshold level of an individual (see 5.1.2).

Note 3: prior to 1988, the basis of bone-conduction calibration was entirely different. Equipment calibrated to the former standard BS 2497 Part 4 (now withdrawn) in terms of vibratory acceleration will give results differing up to 6 dB or more compared with the current standard, in the direction of creating an artificial air–bone gap, or inflating a genuine one.

4.5.3 Procedures

Distinctions have to be made between full-scale calibrations, periodical re-calibrations and routine checks of performance. It is good practice to have the audiometers adjusted at the time of the initial or first re-calibration to give true readings (thus avoiding systematic errors, the use of correction charts etc.), and thereafter to monitor the instrument periodically to ensure that it remains within a specified margin of its last full-scale calibration. It cannot be assumed that a calibration will remain valid for an extended period (years); the transducers (earphones and vibrator) in particular are liable to change through mishandling or electrical overload.

A three-tier system of checks and calibrations evolved for the above purposes is outlined below. The system was originally devised by the former DHSS Advisory Committee on Audiological Equipment (ACAE) in the late 1970s and was subsequently published by the National Physical Laboratory (Shipton, 1987). It was adopted with some modification by ISO in 1989 and the salient points recommended by the present Working Group are summarized below.

Stage A – routine checking and subjective tests. The purpose is to ensure, as far as possible, that the equipment is working properly, that its acoustic output has not noticeably altered and that its attachments, leads and accessories are free from any defect that might upset the test results. The routine checks should be carried out on each day that the equipment is in use for the purpose of medicolegal audiometry. Measuring instruments are not needed for Stage A, but an overall check is made by carrying out a low-intensity listening check under the normal working conditions of the audiometer and test room. This entails sweeping through all appropriate frequencies at a hearing level of 10 dB or 15 dB and listening for 'just audible' tones. The check must be performed by a person with normal, or better than normal, hearing. It should be performed for both earphones as well as the bone vibrator. The following routines should precede the above checks on each occasion that they are performed. Equipment must be left switched on for the recommended warm-up time before use. On battery-powered equipment the state of the battery must be checked. The subject's signalling system must be checked for correct operation.

In addition to the above checks, it is good practice to supplement them periodically (e.g. weekly or fortnightly) with a more formal subjective check. For this purpose a complete a-c audiogram should be carried out with the aid of an assistant, under the normal working conditions of the audiometer and test room; the test person should be one with normal, or better than normal, hearing who is employed consistently over a period of time to develop a running audiogram. The advantages of this procedure are (a) the test will exactly resemble that in normal use and will reveal possible audible malfunctions (e.g. hums or clicks), and (b) the running audiogram data will serve as evidence of quality control.

Stage B – periodic objective checks. This tier checks a number of functions of the audiometer: frequencies of the tones; sound pressure levels in an acoustic coupler or artificial ear, as appropriate; vibratory force levels on a mechanical coupler; levels of the masking noise; attenuator steps; harmonic distortion. The intervals between these checks may be determined by experience but should normally not exceed one year. Changes of sound or vibration output levels of 2 dB or more at any frequency should signal that a complete re-calibration (Stage C) is due. The value of that tier depends upon keeping a proper record of the Stage B checks and any action taken as a result of them.

Note 1: the above guidance on intervals between Stage B checks depends upon the consistent application of Stage A checks.

Note 2: stage B checks require access to at least the following equipment: sound level meter Type 1 complying with BS 5969 or BS 6698; one-third octave band filter set complying with BS 2475; acoustic coupler and/or artificial ear, and mechanical coupler, as described in 4.4; digital frequency counter; oscilloscope; low-noise measuring amplifier (to enable the audiometer hearing level control steps to be checked down to –10 dB HL).

Stage C – baseline calibration. This tier is brought into play at three points: (i) for newly acquired or modified apparatus (including the test room), (ii) when Stage A or Stage B checks have shown up a fault which cannot be rectified without full workshop facilities, and (iii) when, after a long period of time, it is suspected that the equipment may no longer be performing fully to specification. Examples of (iii) might be a suspicion that the masking noise character has changed or that the rise and fall times at the start and finish of each signal may have gone out of specification. Stage C checks and calibrations need not be employed on a routine basis if Stage A and Stage B checks are performed regularly.

Certification. The high standards of audiometric accuracy needed for purposes of disability assessment require that at least the Stage C calibrations of the apparatus (or, in the case of the test room, its qualification of suitability for purpose) be certificated by a competent organization, such as a NAMAS-accredited testing laboratory.

4.6 Background noise requirements for the test room

A quiet environment is essential for accurate audiometry. For air-conduction testing, the headphones provide some measure of exclusion of residual noise in the test room, but this is not the case for bone conduction, where the ear canal is uncovered. Theoretically, therefore, it is the latter case which is crucial. However, this is not necessarily the case in practice, because bone-conduction measurements usually assume importance only when there is at least a small amount of conductive hearing loss, in which case the conductive loss tends to offset the loss of noise exclusion when the ear is uncovered.

Standards exist (BS 6655; ISO 8253-1) for the upper permissible limits of acceptable background noise for audiometry, and these are conditioned by four factors: (a) the lowest hearing threshold level which it is necessary to measure (remembering that the range of normal hearing of young persons extends at least down to –10 dB HL), (b) the acceptable margin by which the selected lowest level may be in error as a direct result of masking of the test tone by the background noise, (c) the lowest test frequency to be measured, and (d) whether or not headphones are in place, and if so what allowance can be made for their sound attenuation.

Desirably the test environment should comply with the above-mentioned standards. However, these standards provide for audiometry over a wider frequency range than that required here. A review of the standards, and an adaptation which is slightly less demanding, is described in Robinson (in press) and is deemed acceptable for present purposes. Recommended noise limits for use in the present context are given in 4.6.1.

> Note: it is necessary to provide for measurement of hearing threshold levels at least down to 0 dB HL, to provide a safety margin for cases of mild, but potentially compensable, disability, and to assist in the detection of spurious hearing threshold level (see 6.1) on the part of otherwise normal claimants.

Qualification of test rooms with respect to background noise requires acoustic expertise, and the resources of specialized equipment not normally available in audiological clinics.

4.6.1 Specific recommendations applicable to audiometry for disability assessment

If the conditions specified in BS 6655 or ISO 8253-1 are not met by the available test facilities, it is nevertheless possible to satisfy the requirements of pure-tone audiometry for disability assessment if the background noise level is within the limits set out in Table 4.1. The main, but not the only, reason why these values are less stringent is the restricted frequency range (1, 2 and 3 kHz only) over which a specified accuracy has to be guaranteed. The conditions applicable to these more relaxed values are given in the footnotes to the table and further described in 5.2.2.

Summary of chapter recommendations

- Equipment for audiometry should comply with BS 5966 with a direct link to national standards for hearing levels.

Table 4.1 Maximum acceptable levels for background noise in the audiometry test room under specified conditions (see footnotes to the table).

Centre frequency of one-third octave band (kHz)	One-third octave band sound pressure level (dB re 20 μPa)	
	Air conduction only[1]	Bone conduction[2]
0.0315	94	97
0.04	89	92
0.05	84	87
0.063	80	82
0.08	75	77
0.1	71	72
0.125	66	66
0.16	62	61
0.2	58	56
0.25	52	50
0.315	47	45
0.4	43	40
0.5	38	34
0.63	33	27
0.8	27	21
1.0	23	16
1.25	25	16
1.6	27	17
2.0	30	17
2.5	32	15
3.15	34	13
4.0	36	11
5.0	35	13
6.3	34	18
8.0	33	24

[1] Valid for air-conduction audiometry only: (a) at frequencies of 1 kHz and above; (b) when typical supra-aural earphones are worn (see 4.1); and (c) for measurements down to 0 dB HL.

[2] Valid for bone-conduction audiometry at frequencies of 1 kHz and above. These values differ from those required solely for air-conduction measurements on the same ears, because they necessarily exclude any allowance for the noise attenuation provided by wearing supra-aural earphones. However, a small upward adjustment of the acceptable noise levels has been included, the effect of which may be a slight underestimation of the magnitude of the air-bone gap. This underestimation could only arise in the case of small overall hearing losses (air-conduction HTLs less than about 10 dB); in such cases, avoidance of error due to background noise masking would necessitate reducing each of the one-third octave band sound pressure levels in this column by 5 dB.

- The use of noise-excluding earphone enclosures is not recommended.
- It is the responsibility of the medical examiner to ensure appropriate quality assurance, including adequate audiometer calibration.
- Background noise levels for audiometry should preferably meet the requirements of BS 6655, but will be acceptable for measurements at 1, 2 and 3 kHz if they meet the relaxed requirements given in Table 4.1.

Chapter 5
Determination of hearing threshold levels in usual cases

5.1 Audiometric procedure

There are different ways of using an audiometer to measure hearing thresholds. For the purposes of hearing disability assessment, uniformity of practice is necessary in order to avoid systematic differences introduced by the method. Provided the recommended procedures are strictly adhered to and the presence of SHTL (see 6.1) is not in question, the methods described below have been proven to give reliable and reasonably reproducible results, and should normally be used. If any variations of these procedures are employed, for example in specialist centres with particular expertise in audiometry, the results are to be adjusted (as appropriate) to accord with the results that would be obtained by the specified procedures.

Note: in case of discordant results from different centres or on different occasions, full details of the audiometric techniques employed and other aspects of quality assurance should be made available to persons directly concerned.

5.1.1 Procedure for air-conduction testing

The procedure should follow the published recommendations of the BSA and BAOL (Anon, 1981) and should include repeats at the frequencies 1, 2 and 3 kHz (see 5.2.3.1, which also indicates how to deal with results that do not agree). The BSA/BAOL recommendations describe two equivalent methods of conducting manual audiometry, referred to as Methods A and B.

Note 1: method A is a '10 dB down, –5 dB up' paradigm, in which multiple ascents are made with single stimulus presentations. Threshold is taken to be the lowest level at which two or more positive responses are given in at least half of the series of ascents. Method B is a variant, using 5-dB steps (up and down) in which multiple presentations are given at each level to establish the lowest level for which at least two positive responses out of a possible four are obtained. Various refinements and simplified versions of the procedures are described in the reference.

Masking, where appropriate, should follow the recommendations published by BSA in 1986.

Note 2: the guidelines given in the above references for obtaining and interpreting responses to the tone stimuli should be followed precisely, or as closely as individual circumstances permit, in order to avoid rounding up to the next higher step of hearing level.

5.1.2 *Procedure for bone-conduction testing*

For the purposes of disability assessment, bone-conduction testing needs to be carried out on both sides, with masking routinely applied to the non-test ear (irrespective of which is the better ear) at 35 dB SL, and at such other levels as may be needed to define any masking plateau at higher levels (see Note 1 below). The vibrator should be applied to the mastoid prominence contralateral to the masking transducer, first one way round and then the other. Tone presentations should follow the same method, A or B (see above) as used for the air-conduction testing, and appropriate additional masking levels should be used according to the plateau-seeking method recommended by the BSA (1985). Note 2 of 5.1.1 also applies to bone-conduction testing.

Note 1: the above exception to the BSA recommendations should be noted with respect to the masking. The BSA rules on when to apply masking are intended for clinical diagnostic purposes and are not appropriate for quantitative compensation assessment which requires identical procedures to be followed on both sides. The reason for the exception is to ensure that the small but distinct central masking effect of contralaterally applied noise on the observed thresholds applies equally to both ears, and also because this procedure corresponds to the conditions underlying the standard reference zero.

Note 2: recommendations were published by BSA in 1985 for bone-conduction testing without masking (BSA, 1985) which are relevant in part. In particular, the appendix to those recommendations draws attention to certain technical pitfalls in bone-conduction testing.

Note 3: the technique of bone-conduction testing with masking for use in the medicolegal context, described by Coles et al. (1991), is also recommended as a way of meeting all the above requirements without being unduly time-consuming.

5.1.3 *Reporting the results of audiometry*

The quantities to be specified for the disability assessment procedure described in this Report are the hearing threshold levels, by air and bone conduction, at 1, 2 and 3 kHz only. The audiometric results should be expressed as hearing levels at individual frequencies to the nearest 5-dB step, using the format and symbols for pure-tone audiograms published by the BSA in 1989.

Note: complete air-conduction audiograms (0.25–8 kHz) will be required for the purposes of diagnosis, but the test conditions specified here will not necessarily guarantee accurate results at frequencies outside the range 1 to 3 kHz (especially at low frequencies).

The following additional technical data should be included in the medicolegal report (see Chapter 11):

- Type(s) of audiometer used
- Type(s) of earphone and bone vibrator used
- The audiometric standard(s) to which the results are referred
- Identification of last certificate (or other evidence) of calibration
- Method of audiometry employed (in sufficient detail)
- Types of noise, transducer and technique used for masking
- Which background noise criteria have been complied with, for air- and bone-conduction tests.

5.2 Sources of error in audiometry

A distinction has to be made between systematic effects (which affect the accuracy of a measurement) and random uncertainties (which affect its repeatability). Both are sources of error but are distinguished by their differing natures: systematic effects can in principle be allowed for and the associated error cancelled by appropriate corrections (although this is not always feasible), whereas random uncertainties can only be reduced by averaging repeat measurements and can never be eliminated entirely. Both systematic and random effects occur to an important extent in audiometry, and both are present in the objective as well as the subjective aspects of the measurements. The principal points to watch in connection with audiometry where quantitative accuracy is of prime importance are outlined below.

5.2.1 Sources of objective error

The main sources of systematic error are as follows:

- Calibration error of the audiometer. The standard specifications for audiometers (e.g. BS 5966) are manufacturing specifications in which the various functions are required to perform within specified tolerances of specified nominal values. Thus, for example, an instrument stated to conform to specification may deliver sound pressure levels within ± 3 dB of the proper values corresponding to the dial settings. By contrast, a calibration consists of a determination of the actual levels, frequencies etc., that the instrument delivers, and (desirably) an adjustment of its preset controls to bring these values into exact alignment with the nominal values. A statement that an instrument conforms to the standard is a necessary but insufficient condition for correct performance.
- Effect of earphone type. Audiometric standards are drawn up in such a way as to allow the use of earphones of varying patterns (but not an unlimited variety), each with its own set of reference equivalent threshold sound pressure levels. Whichever pattern is used, the same average hearing threshold levels will be obtained (save for residual imperfections in the standards) if a large and constant group of subjects is tested. This, however, does not apply to each individual because of unpredictable interactions between the acoustic characteristics of individual ears and different types of earphone. It is therefore best to restrict the type of earphone to those which are in most general use (in practice, the Telephonics Corporation TDH series).

- Accuracy of the tone frequencies. Standard hearing threshold levels can be obtained only at the frequencies specified in the standards of audiometric zero (which include 1, 2 and 3 kHz). If the apparatus produces tones appreciably different from the nominal values, the resulting measurements can be in error from three causes: (a) the ear is being tested at the wrong frequency (this may be a major effect if the threshold of the ear under test has a strong frequency dependence, such as a 'ski-slope' or a marked fine-frequency ripple in the neighbourhood of the test frequency); (b) the normal threshold of hearing could differ appreciably from the audiometric zero at the nominal frequency (this difference being a property of the average human ear), thus causing the hearing level control to deliver spurious sound or vibration levels; and (c) if the frequency has shifted from its last calibration value, the frequency response of the earphone may cause an incorrect sound pressure level to be developed (this problem relates mainly to high frequencies and is unlikely to cause serious error at 1, 2 or 3 kHz).

5.2.2 *Systematic and random uncertainties associated with audiometric technique*

A miscellany of effects falls under this heading:

- Background noise in the test room. Minimum requirements for admissible background noise are set out in 4.6.1. The limiting noise levels in the table were arrived at on the basis that continuous noise, the spectrum of which does not exceed the specified values in any one-third octave band, will cause a threshold shift not exceeding 2 dB at any of the key test frequencies (1, 2, 3 kHz) when measuring air-conduction thresholds down to 0 dB HL. This does not necessarily mean that the background noise is itself inaudible to the subject – only that it will not interfere with the test by more than the error criterion of 2 dB. There is not a simple relation between noise level and the error it causes. For example, to ensure an error not exceeding 1 dB, all noise levels in the tables would have to be 5 dB lower. Conversely, if an error not exceeding 5 dB were to be tolerated, the levels could theoretically be set 8 dB higher; however, an error of this magnitude is unacceptably large.
- Fitting the headphones and bone vibrator. Assuming that the headband is already adjusted to provide the correct force of application, it will nevertheless be true that the sound pressure or vibratory force (as the case may be) delivered by the transducer does not repeat exactly on successive placements. Uncertainty in positioning the transducers on the head gives rise to an ineradicable source of random error in audiometry. It is more severe in the case of the vibrator than of the earphone. Fortunately, the effect is least for middle frequencies (including 1, 2 and 3 kHz). Nevertheless, the audiometrician should take steps to minimize the uncertainty by careful placement of the transducers, and by ensuring that they are not moved (accidentally or deliberately) during the course of testing. Accoutrements such as spectacle frames and head ornaments should be removed, and care taken that superfluous hair is not entrapped by the earphone cushion. In bone-conduction

audiometry, it is important to ensure that the vibrator makes contact only at the intended point (over the mastoid prominence), and that its headband makes no mechanical contact with the (separate) headband when one is used to support a supra-aural masking earphone on the other side.

- Signalling system. The subject's response to stimuli is best communicated by means of a press button. This should be silent in operation, with a positive 'feel', but not so stiff as to fatigue the finger.
- Miscellaneous noise. Clothes rub of the transducer cables is to be avoided; also, the seat should be reasonably comfortable though firm and free from creaks.
- Stimulus presentation. Initial familiarization, the preferred order of frequencies, the duration of on- and off-periods etc. are described in the BSA and BAOL recommendations referred to in 5.1.1 and 5.1.2, and should be closely adhered to.
- Alternative modes of audiometry. Some audiometers provide an automated sequence of signal presentations, simulating manual methods of audiometry. Some other computer-controlled types go further in providing a time-optimized sequence and algorithmic computation of the thresholds. These instruments may yield results systematically shifted with respect to the manual methods A and B recommended here, and details of their performance (with corrections if necessary) should be provided (see 5.1). Despite their several advantages in other applications, audiometers providing only fixed-frequency self-recording are not recommended for present purposes, principally because they are not normally adaptable to the required bone-conduction testing. If, in exceptional cases, such equipment is used for air-conduction testing, the results read from the self-recorded traces in the manner specified in BS 6655 have to be adjusted. This adjustment specified in BS 6655 as +3 dB is to be added to self-recorded hearing threshold levels. The result is then rounded to the nearest 5 dB (see Example 2 in Appendix A).

5.2.3 *Uncertainties associated with the subject*

5.2.3.1 Normal expectation of audiometric reliability. Factors affecting performance in audiometry have been fully reviewed by Stephens (1981). In Table 15.1 of the reference, he lists 38 sources of variance in audiometric testing. The sources attributable to the subject being tested include motivation, comprehension of instructions, judgmental criteria, detection variance, learning effect, personality, circadian effects, attention, fatigue, colds, wax, temporary effects of preceding noise exposure, and real fluctuation in hearing sensitivity.

Many of the above factors are outside the control of the tester, but attention is needed to the following. Ensuring that instructions are understood and that the subject is attentive depends on observation of the claimant's performance during audiometry and, if comprehension or attention is lacking or suspected, it should be corrected by immediate re-instruction. Enquiry should be made as to whether or not the claimant has a cold and whether or not this, or any other temporary factor, seems to be affecting the hearing or quality of performance. Enquiry is also needed as to the nature, loudness and duration of any occupational or other noise exposure in the preceding 24 hours, together with notes on any hearing protector worn in that period. The ears should be examined for wax and any other factor possibly associated with a temporary effect on hearing. History, or other diagnostic evidence, of any factors possibly associated with a real fluctuation in hearing sensitivity should also be sought.

Assuming that there are no such temporary influences on hearing, and that there is no SHTL (see 6.1), there remain variations which are inseparable from the process of audiometry, but which become apparent only if the measurements are repeated. From the many experimental studies on this subject, the following conclusions can be distilled (Robinson, 1991a): (a) repeatability varies greatly from person to person but no test has yet been devised to separate 'sheep' from 'goats' in this respect in advance of repeat measurements; (b) repeatability is best at 1 and 2 kHz and poorer outside these limits especially at 6 kHz; (c) different audiometric techniques (e.g. manual, self-recording or microprocessor-controlled) can produce systematic differences of measured HTL (see, for example, 5.2.2) but there is little to choose between them in respect of repeatability; (d) with 5-dB steps and the frequencies relevant to disability assessment (1, 2, 3 kHz), the most prevalent (modal) difference between occasions will be ± 5 dB, and the number of zero differences will exceed the number of differences of ± 10 dB or greater; (e) a proportion of subjects will exhibit repeatability worse than ± 10 dB at one or more individual frequency, but very few will yield consistently poor results at all frequencies tested; (f) repeats at 1, 2 or 3 kHz, even over an extended period of time (months), worse than ± 20 dB can be virtually ruled out, save for an occasional freak result due to some adventitious circumstance; (g) where only a single measurement is made on a given ear, errors of the above magnitudes will inevitably go undetected.

In view of (g) above, there is a strong case for repeating audiometry routinely and recording both results. This practice is recommended, at least in the case of air conduction at the key frequencies of 1, 2 and 3 kHz, taking the step of removing and replacing the earphones between repeats. Where such repeats differ by 5 dB the lower (more acute) threshold should be taken, and if the difference is 10 dB the average should be taken; these rules implement the principle of taking the average result and rounding down to the nearest 5 dB, in recognition of the essentially asymmetrical nature of subjective error in audiometry. In the event of larger differences occurring, the case merits further testing. It should, of course, be appreciated that repeating the audiometry will only reduce the uncertainties of measurement where random factors are at work; the fact that measurements repeat exactly does not necessarily mean that they are true. Even individuals who give spurious results (SHTL) may give perfect repeats.

5.2.3.2 Abnormal performance or unusual occurrences. Some of the factors which may cause the subject to indicate incorrect thresholds are dealt with in 5.2.3.1 above, and SHTL is covered in 6.1. The other fairly common source of error due to the subject arises when the pressure of the audiometric earphone causes the ear canal walls to collapse and thus occlude the ear canal. This is quite likely to occur in the elderly with thin atrophic cartilage of the external ear, in those with narrow ear canals, and in post-traumatic thickening of the external ear near the opening of the ear canal (Coles, 1967). It causes a pseudo-conductive hearing loss, due to obstruction of the ear canal in the a-c tests, but not in b-c. The clue to a collapse of the ear canal is when, in the presence of an apparent air–bone gap, other tests, such as tuning forks or immittance audiometry, provide no supporting evidence of a conductive hearing loss. The proof of the diagnosis, and the means of obtaining genuine HTLs, is to insert a firm tube (e.g. an aural impedance-testing tip) into the ear canal, and then to retest the a-c thresholds.

5.2.4 *Effects associated with the audiometrician and the interpretation of responses*

The audiometrician can influence test results in manual audiometry in several ways, as follows: (a) by using procedures other than those authoritatively recommended (e.g. Anon, 1981; BSA, 1985, 1986), especially in connection with variable lengths of signal and interval, the use of both onset and offset of signal and of response to decide on the acceptability of a response, and the criterion of threshold; (b) by allowing bias to influence judgment of presence or absence of response to a signal and in judgment of a threshold, such bias usually being accidental but potentially influenced by sympathy for or against the claimant, or by preconceived ideas as to his or her hearing ability; (c) by exercising skill, care and knowledge regarding the particular needs in medicolegal cases for accurate b-c threshold measurements (see 5.1.2); (d) by failing to recognize and report unreliability of response and uncertainty of threshold, leading to an unjustifiably firm statement of the threshold measured.

Self-recording audiometry is not subject to procedural error unless some very unusual equipment or technique is used.

5.3 Qualifications and training of personnel

In order to achieve acceptable estimates of hearing disability using the recommendations described in this Report, it is necessary that audiometry is carried out conscientiously and according to the specified procedures. This entails that persons carrying out the audiometry are properly trained and qualified in the task. The methods described in the Report also require that subjects are examined medically with a view to the diagnosis of any hearing disorder. This section sets out to describe the necessary training and/or qualifications for persons undertaking audiometry, but does not attempt to define the required medical training for the medical examiner. However, if audiometry is carried out by medical examiners, they must meet the training and qualification requirements for performing audiometry.

The overall audiometric procedure involves the following: daily Stage A checking of the audiometer and ancillary apparatus (see 4.5.3); informal observation of the communication abilities of the subject; otoscopic examination relevant to audiometry; noting of relevant abnormalities of the ear that might affect the test results; performance of air-conduction and bone-conduction audiometry with masking according to the methods described in 5.1.1 and 5.1.2; recording and interpretation of the test results; understanding of the common sources of error in pure-tone audiometry. The person performing the test must be able to perform all of these tasks and must also possess a basic understanding of hearing and the effects of noise on hearing.

A number of established courses include training on the above topics as part of a more general training to satisfy the requirements of the British Association of Audiology Technicians Part I and Part II examinations or the Hearing Aid Council's examination; there are also MSc and Diploma courses in audiology run by universities in the UK. Persons possessing any of the above qualifications are deemed to be qualified to perform audiometry for disability assessment to the requirements of this Report. In the absence of such qualifications, it is the responsibility of the medical examiner to ensure that the person carrying out the test is competent in the tasks outlined above, in which case the medical examiner must be prepared to provide evidence to that effect if required.

Summary of chapter recommendations

- Basic audiometric testing and reporting of results should follow the methods recommended by the British Society of Audiology.
- Two separate determinations should be made of each of the air-conduction thresholds at 1, 2 and 3 kHz for each ear.
- Testing should be carried out by an appropriately qualified person, as defined in 5.3.

Chapter 6
Determination of hearing threshold levels in special cases

6.1 Detection of spurious hearing threshold level (SHTL)

A spurious hearing threshold level (SHTL) may deviate in either direction from the genuine hearing threshold level (GHTL), but is more often in the direction of greater apparent hearing loss. SHTL may account for all of the apparent hearing loss, but more often it comprises an overlay superimposed on some degree of genuinely abnormal hearing.

The origins of SHTLs are complex and their detection in practice is not a simple process. Inflation of a hearing loss may go undetected even by experienced medical examiners. Unfortunately, the measurement of hearing by means of pure-tone audiometry tends to facilitate such inflation. Many people can be remarkably proficient in simulation or exaggeration of a hearing loss, often with good repeatability of audiometric responses. It is probable that such subjects use a criterion of equal loudness rather than absolute threshold. Thus the tester will need to have recourse to a number of tests in order to detect SHTL and to estimate the GHTL.

The major indicator of SHTL is evidence of intra- and inter-test inconsistencies. People with frequent personal experience of carrying out pure-tone audiometry by manual techniques should be able to sense or observe unusually variable responses. Usually these are due to inattention or inability, but also someone deliberately simulating or exaggerating their hearing impairment will often show such variability. Criteria of undue variability are difficult to define, and would in any event depend on the exact method of test, but the tester should be encouraged to put a note with the audiogram indicating any unusual degree of variability, which may then become an indication for further investigation, for example by cortical electric response audiometry (CERA).

There are a number of special audiometric techniques which purport to enhance the likelihood of SHTL being detected, for example that by Harris (1958). An abbreviated version of this suggested by Kerr et al. (1975) is performed as follows. The threshold at 1 kHz, or at another frequency if more relevant, is tested in descending 10-dB steps starting from 90 dB HL, or greater if needed, until the claimant stops responding. This is followed by an ascending 10-dB step series starting at –10 dB HL until he responds. In cases of SHTL, the descending threshold will often be 10–30 dB poorer than the ascending threshold; that is, there will be an ascending–descending gap in favour of the ascending threshold giving better results whereas in absence of SHTL it usually yields slightly less sensitive thresholds.

Because NIHL usually affects both ears, seldom with large differences between them, the Stenger test is not appropriate for such cases. But in head or ear injury claimants, the hearing loss often appears to be unilateral or affecting one ear very much more than the other, and this difference is quite commonly spurious. For such cases the audiometric Stenger test is an extremely effective detector of SHTL, as well as giving a quantitative measure of the genuine left/right difference at the test frequency selected. The reader is referred elsewhere for details of the test procedures (Coles and Priede, 1971; Coles, 1982).

If sweep-frequency self-recording audiometry (SFSRA) is available as an additional test or is used routinely, SHTL can often be detected by considering the relationship of self-recorded thresholds using pulsed and continuous tone stimuli respectively, as well as from the general features of the response. SHTL is not necessarily associated with a 'continuous-better-than-pulsed' threshold; other patterns may occur. This is partly, but not entirely, due to abnormal auditory adaptation, if present, offsetting any 'Type V' effect. An important feature of SFSRA is that it effectively prevents SHTL arising from observer error or bias, which of course can creep in with manual audiometry, especially when not conducted according to a strict protocol.

In order for claimants with an underlying NIHL to exaggerate their hearing loss, they may use a criterion of equal loudness. Due to recruitment of loudness at the frequencies with true hearing loss, the audiometric contour tends to progressively flatten according to the degree of exaggeration; that is, the more it becomes a loudness response rather than a threshold response (see example depicted by Coles and Priede, 1971, and the evidence from CERA tests in such cases given by Coles and Mason, 1984). Thus, a flattened audiogram in cases of suspected NIHL is a feature highly suggestive of SHTL, and CERA has been recommended in such cases whenever the apparent a-c threshold at 0.5 kHz exceeds 35 dB (Alberti et al., 1978) or 25 dB (Coles, 1982). The latter criterion should be adopted.

A comparison of thresholds measured by a-c and b-c testing can also be useful in the detection of SHTL. When b-c thresholds are appreciably better than the corresponding a-c thresholds, this is usually taken as indicating the presence of CHL, but it may in fact result from spurious measurements. Such an apparent difference in thresholds (generally referred to as an air–bone gap if in this direction) does not necessarily imply the existence of a conductive hearing loss. Moreover, a conductive loss may arise from a disorder of the middle ear or may be a pseudo-conductive loss due to ear canal collapse (see 5.2.3.2). Furthermore, middle-ear, spurious and pseudo-conductive losses may coexist in varying degrees. To elucidate this complexity the examiner may need to have recourse to the results of a variety of other tests. It should be noted that similarity of the a-c and b-c thresholds does not of itself exclude SHTL, because of individuals using a loudness criterion. It is also extremely unlikely that a genuine full audiogram would show no difference at all between a-c and b-c thresholds at any frequency.

Inspection of the claimant's audiogram will suggest the degree of auditory disability that the individual might reasonably be expected to have. If there is inconsistency here with informal observations of the claimant's evident hearing ability/disability, the examiner should suspect SHTL.

If facilities for speech audiometry are available, it is recommended to apply the methods described by Coles and Priede (1976) or Fournier (1956). These will give a more accurate quantification of speech hearing ability although losing the advantage of informality. If the speech recognition threshold level relative to the normal biological baseline is more than about 10 dB better than the average of the best two pure-tone thresholds, SHTL can be suspected; if more than about 20 dB better, SHTL is almost certain.

Cortical electric response audiometry is a method for detecting and quantifying SHTL. However, it is not infallible and cannot replace methods of behavioural audiometry, particularly because the information it can give on frequencies above 4 kHz is of limited value. Another feature is that CERA, unless declared to be a routine test for all claimants, is psychologically intrusive because claimants submitted to this test frequently realize that the medical examiner suspects them of malingering. Nevertheless, this is not considered to be a serious objection to using it when indicated.

6.2 Estimation of genuine hearing threshold level (GHTL) in the presence of SHTL

Occasionally, the Stenger test or speech audiometry will indicate thresholds in the region of zero (i.e. normal hearing) which can therefore be taken as the GHTL. More often these tests will merely indicate or suggest the presence of SHTL, and also that the GHTL is not greater than some level shown by that test. For these cases, it is necessary to carry out CERA. Often, at any one sitting, this has to be limited to between four and eight tests (e.g. two to four frequencies in each ear) because of the time required which is associated with a deterioration in response, and to tests in the 0.5–4 kHz range. Tests at 6 and 8 kHz can also be attempted, but only if responses at all lower frequencies have been well defined.

Very occasionally, CERA cannot be performed at all; for example, when subjects keep falling asleep or when they persistently fidget or make muscle contractions. The latter behaviour is sometimes deliberate, to foil the test: if this is suspected, the facts of the situation and careful observation of the behaviour of the claimant should be reported in detail.

The results of CERA usually lead to one of four interpretations. These are based on the subjective/objective difference; that is, the behavioural threshold minus CERA threshold, averaged over those frequencies that have been tested by both methods (Coles and Mason, 1984).

- Occasionally the average difference is less than −10 dB, in which case the CERA results should be discarded as being less sensitive than the behavioural test results.
- If the average difference is in the range ±10 dB, the behavioural audiogram can be taken as corroborated by the CERA tests and the overall assessment should be based on the former.
- If the average difference lies in the range +11 to +15 dB, there is strong suspicion of SHTL and another CERA test may be required, which preferably should be carried out at another centre and without knowledge of the previous results.

- If the average difference is more than +15 dB, there is a high probability of SHTL. In absence of convincing evidence to the contrary (e.g. from at least two other CERA audiograms) the CERA thresholds should then be taken as the definitive ones for disability assessment, without making any correction for any supposed insensitivity of CERA. Of course that leaves a diagnostic problem, but often there remains sufficient evidence for a diagnostic opinion to be given, or further evidence can be obtained, for example from repeat behavioural tests after explanation and reinstruction.

Summary of chapter recommendations

- When there is any indication of spurious hearing threshold levels, as defined in 6.1, cortical electric response audiometry should be applied and interpreted as described in 6.2.

Chapter 7
Evaluation of attributable and constitutional components

7.1 Principles of evaluation

As a general principle, attributable disability will be arrived at by first evaluating the overall disability corresponding to the actual hearing loss and then subtracting from this the disability which could be ascribed solely to the constitutional part, or parts, of the hearing loss (see definitions in Chapter 2). The following sections deal with the components of hearing threshold level associated with age (AAHL) and with conductive hearing loss (CHL) respectively. Determination of the notional disability due to a constitutional component, or combination of constitutional components, of the hearing threshold level is described in 9.1.2.

> Note: in most cases, CHL is a non-compensable component, but occasionally it is the CHL itself which is compensable. In such circumstances, the procedures given in 7.5.2 would apply equally well to the assessment of the amount of CHL as a compensable disorder.

7.2 Evaluation of the decibel value of age-associated hearing loss

For any individual above the age of about 25, some element of AAHL will most probably be present, but it can only be measured when other components of SNHL are known to be absent. This, however, will not be the case with claimants, in the nature of things. Consequently, for the purposes of disability assessment, a notional attribution of AAHL according to age is unavoidable. For this Report, the median value for the appropriate sex is used as this notional value, based on ISO 7029 which defines the expected distributions of hearing threshold levels (HTL) for otologically normal males and females as a function of age. The function has different parameters for each audiometric frequency and for each sex. Only the median HTLs at 1, 2 and 3 kHz are of interest here. The age range for which ISO 7029 is applicable is from 18 to 70 years inclusive.

Table A1 in Annex A gives the median HTLs *summed* over 1, 2 and 3 kHz for males and females between the ages of 18 and 80 years, to be used to allow for AAHL in this Report. For this purpose, ISO 7029 has been extrapolated beyond its stated scope to include subjects with ages between 71 and 80 years, and the data for the extended age range are shown in italics. When the extended range of AAHL has been used for a particular assessment, the medical examiner should qualify his report accordingly.

7.3 Mandatory requirements

There are five main requirements for the evaluation of attributable hearing loss, as follows:

- Measurement of the pure-tone air-conduction hearing threshold levels.
- Diagnosis of its probable cause(s). This will include the taking of a full medical and occupational history, obtaining a description of the effects of the hearing loss and/or tinnitus on the claimant, clinical examination of the claimant, and consideration of the air-conduction audiogram in terms of degree and configuration of hearing losses in each ear. Bone-conduction audiometry will also be required in most cases. Note that diagnoses will quite often have to include conductive or sensorineural hearing loss of unknown origin.
- Quantification of the overall hearing impairment and disability, and an assessment of handicap and of any tinnitus.
- Estimation of any constitutional impairment and disability, and thence of the ***attributable disability***, which is the disability attributable to the alleged injury or disease and to any other injuries or diseases of like nature (usually noise- or injury-induced, both compensable and non-compensable).
- Apportionment of the attributable disability into its allegedly compensable and non-compensable components.

7.4 Conditional and discretionary tests

Additional tests which may be necessary or additionally helpful include the following:

- Indicator tests for spurious hearing threshold level (SHTL) and measurement tests for the genuine hearing threshold level (GHTL), as outlined in Chapter 6. SHTL may also be indicated by the following two items when compared with the pure-tone audiogram.
- Tympanometry, complete with measurements of the acoustic reflexes to show their presence or absence, character, threshold and decay. These will help to corroborate or argue against presence of any conductive hearing loss, and yield other diagnostic information in addition to being a useful indicator test for SHTL.
- Speech audiometry. This may add further information on possible disability and rehabilitational limitations, in addition to being a useful indicator test for SHTL.
- Measurements of the most comfortable loudness level and of the threshold of uncomfortable loudness, which may indicate hyperacusis and/or rehabilitational limitations.
- Tinnitus tests (see C1 in Appendix C) to give some indication of the pitch and loudness of the tinnitus and perhaps also its maskability.
- Vestibular function tests and auditory brainstem evoked responses, and perhaps imaging and haematological tests, for differential diagnostic purposes.

7.5 Evaluation of a conductive component of hearing loss

7.5.1 Relevant conductive hearing loss (CHL)

The relevant conductive loss element is that which, if present, can be positively attributed to a disorder of the middle ear. Evaluation of this component is based upon the difference between the hearing threshold levels (HTL) by air and bone conduction respectively, viz. the air–bone gap (ABG). However, the CHL is not in general equal in magnitude to the ABG, for the reason described in 7.5.2(ii).

Note: in some cases a secondary cochlear component may be present. This takes the form of a sensorineural loss consequent upon the existence of a primary middle-ear disorder. Where the conductive disorder is non-compensable, this secondary loss will form a non-compensable component of the overall sensorineural loss, which also contains the essential compensable element. The amount of secondary sensorineural loss is highly variable and depends upon the nature of the primary middle-ear disorder. However, this component does not easily lend itself to quantitative evaluation. For the purposes of this Report, secondary sensorineural involvement will be deemed to be absent unless there is convincing evidence to the contrary. Clinical examination (e.g. fistula sign), radiology of the internal ear, and history of ear surgery or suggestive of suppurative labyrinthitis or of erosion of the labyrinth may provide such evidence. Additional evidence may be found in the claimant's medical records, perhaps indicating conditions or complications likely to affect the internal ear or providing evidence of the progression of the hearing disorder, and also in the audiometric pattern and amount of a-c and b-c hearing loss, comparing between a-c and b-c and between the two ears. Where there is such evidence, this sensorineural component will constitute another identifiable (non-compensable or compensable) component of the overall hearing loss for which an arbitrary adjustment may be appropriate, the amount of such adjustment being at the medical examiner's discretion.

7.5.2 Evaluation of the decibel value of the CHL

The quantitative procedure for evaluating CHL is described in (i) and (iii) below. The rationale for this procedure is outlined in (ii).

(i) The measurements from which CHL is to be evaluated are the HTLs by air conduction and bone conduction, in each ear, averaged over the frequencies 1, 2 and 3 kHz only, and measured in accordance with the procedures described in 5.1.1 and 5.1.2 respectively. Each ear is to be considered separately. The algebraic difference between the averages for air and bone conduction respectively is the air–bone gap (ABG) expressed in decibels.

(ii) It must be appreciated that the ABG, as defined in (i), does not directly measure the amount of transmission loss of the middle ear. There are two reasons for this (which are in addition to any measurement error).

First, in the case of young otologically normal persons without any hearing loss, there are statistical variations of both the air-conduction and bone-conduction thresholds either side of the average values which, by definition, are zero for both measures. Likewise, the difference (i.e. the ABG) also varies around a mean value of zero, the observed standard deviation of the ABG for the three-frequency average HTL being of the order 5–6 dB. A large part of this variability arises from individual differences in the acoustical and mechanical parameters of ears and skulls. These anatomical variations are not, of course, confined to young otologically normal persons, but apply generally, and they give rise to an ineradicable uncertainty in the measurement of individual air–bone gaps.

Secondly, where a conductive loss due to a middle-ear disorder is present, the measured bone-conduction threshold is artificially raised (due to the so-called Carhart effect). This has the tendency to yield an underestimate of the true conductive loss. A qualitative explanation is that obstruction of the middle ear, for whatever reason, not only creates the conductive loss (the true magnitude of which it is desired to evaluate), but also affects two of the three pathways by which externally applied cranial vibrations are transmitted to the cochlea. In normal ears, the Carhart effect is absent, but as a conductive loss increases to the point where these pathways are virtually obliterated the Carhart effect gradually increases from zero to a limiting value (of the order 15 dB for the three-frequency average). The course of the Carhart effect between zero and its limiting value is indeterminate. Furthermore, the limiting value is not identical for all individuals.

There are two implications of these phenomena:

- Anatomical variations between individuals mean that positive values of the ABG exceeding 10 dB will be quite common, even in the complete absence of conductive loss, and these will be matched by correspondingly common occurrences of –10 dB and even more negative values. Values outside the range ± 15 dB will also occur occasionally without their being clinically significant; however, these are sufficiently rare that, as a working rule, values of ABG exceeding +15 dB will be deemed to signify the undoubted presence of an element of conductive loss. Conservatively, ABG values of +15 dB and below (including negative values) are deemed to be not significant for compensation purposes, even though this does not exclude the possibility of there being some conductive loss in some cases. These values apply to audiometry carefully conducted to the strict rules described above (see 4.5.2 and 5.1.2).
- When the measured ABG is positive and large enough to indicate the undoubted presence of CHL, the true magnitude of such loss will be larger (by the amount of the Carhart effect) than might appear from the observed value of the ABG. This, however, has to be offset by the fact that the ABG is subject to the (indeterminate) uncertainty discussed above. In practice, therefore, it is only possible to assert that the CHL in such cases exceeds the value (ABG – 15) dB.

(iii) The phenomena described in (ii) above are taken into account, in a simplified manner and as a reasonable compromise, to define a relation to be used for determining the amount of CHL of the ear in question. The relation is as shown in Table 7.1.

Table 7.1 Magnitude of conductive hearing loss (CHL) to be used for assessment as a function of the measured air–bone gap (ABG).

Range of measured ABG *averaged over* 1–2–3 kHz (dB)	Amount of CHL *summed over* 1–2–3 kHz (dB)
+15 and below (including negative values)	Nil
Between 15 and 30	6 x (ABG −15)
30 and over	3 x ABG

Note: the values in the second column are given in the form required for the evaluation described in 9.2.2.

The simplifications inherent in the above relations rest upon two opposing influences: (a) the Carhart effect, which is assumed to increase linearly with CHL until it attains its limiting value of 15 dB when the true CHL is 30 dB; (b) the uncertainties of magnitude of the ABG (due both to the inherent statistical variations and to measurement errors), which are accommodated by subtracting 15 dB from the measured value of ABG.

> Note: the repeated occurrences of 15 dB in (a) and (b) are unrelated; the fact that they are numerically equal (to the nearest 5 dB) is simply a coincidence.

Summary of chapter recommendations

- The general principle of assessment of attributable disability is to evaluate the overall disability and then to subtract the notional disability due to the constitutional components alone.
- The notional disability due to constitutional components is obtained by converting the notional hearing threshold level due to those components into disability. (The method for combining the notional components of HTL is given in 9.2.)
- Estimation of conductive hearing loss from measurement of the air–bone gap should take account of the possibility of positive air–bone gaps arising out of biological variation and measurement uncertainty. A specific rule for determining the conductive hearing loss to be used in assessment calculations is given in Table 7.1.

Chapter 8
Tables for calculating percentage disability

8.1 Source material and derivation

An outline of the methods used hitherto for assessing disability from the hearing threshold levels is given in Chapter 3. Few previous methods can claim to have attempted to determine the required relationship in a satisfactory quantitative manner, and most owe more to intuition than to scientific method. Relevant data for this purpose were, however, gathered in the course of the National Study of Hearing (Davis, 1989) carried out by the MRC Institute of Hearing Research. Over 2000 records have been studied in which randomly selected members of the population gave hearing threshold levels coupled with self-ratings of hearing ability on a scale of 0–100. These data have been analysed and presented in mathematical form (Lutman and Robinson, 1992). For the purposes of the present report, the median data from that analysis have been adopted.

8.2 Basic relation between hearing threshold level and percentage disability

The basic relation derived from the above-mentioned analysis applies to persons with approximately equal hearing in both ears, and is expressed in the equations below. The case of unequal ears is handled by an extension described in 8.3.

The average of the HTLs at 1, 2 and 3 kHz, denoted by H_{123}, is related to percentage disability, D, by

$$D = U - 4.08173\exp[0.11712(4.08173 - U)] \qquad \text{Equation 8.1}$$

where

$$U = 100\exp[-\exp(1.05594 - 0.0125309H_{123} - 0.000185186H_{123}^2)] \qquad \text{Equation 8.2}$$

The user of this Report will not need to employ the above equations directly, but simply to use Table A2 of Annex A which has been computed from them.

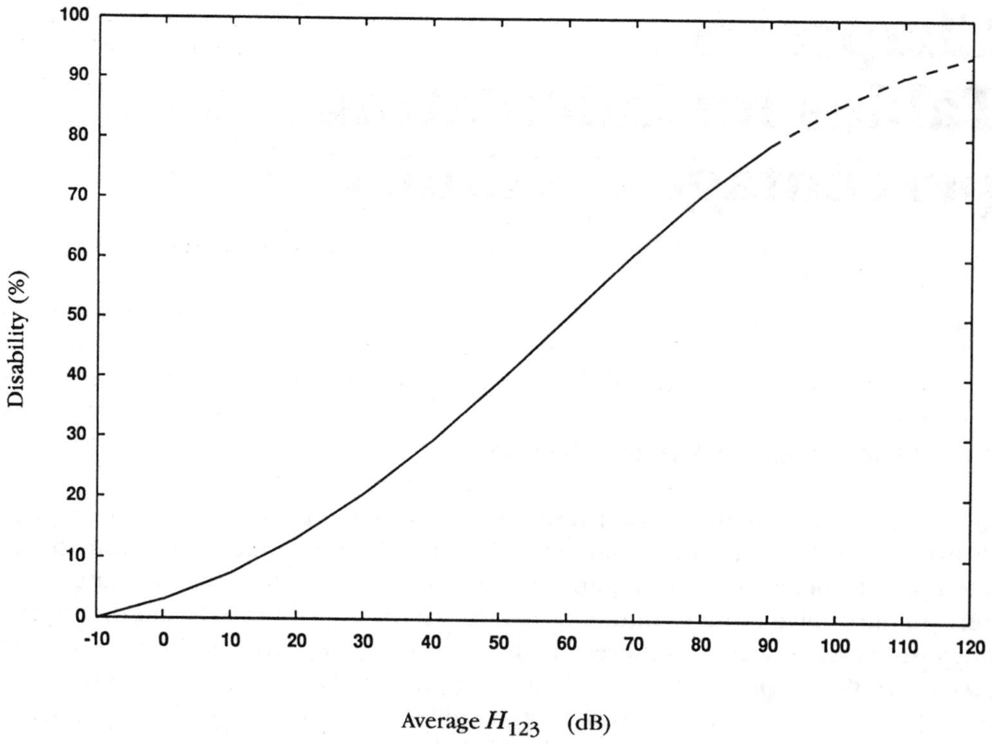

Figure 8.1 Proposed scale relation of hearing disability to hearing impairment based on Lutman and Robinson (1992). Disability is expressed as a percentage. Impairment is expressed as the average of the hearing threshold levels at 1, 2 and 3 kHz measured in the better ear. The function is shown broken for impairments above 90 dB where there was a paucity of data.

The features of the relationship may be seen in Figure 8.1. The growth of D with H_{123} starts at $H_{123} = -10$ dB HL and increases slowly at first, then at a more rapid rate, and finally approaches the upper limit in a long-tailed manner.

Most previous published relationships have assumed the existence of a distinct 'low fence' a value of HTL below which there is zero disability and at which there is a sharp discontinuity followed by a rapid increase in disability with increasing HTL. This kind of relationship is not supported by the experimental evidence referred to in 8.1, which points to a smooth transition from zero to finite values of percentage disability without any discontinuity. Although the rate of increase for individuals could only have been observed if there had been a prospective study covering many years, examination of the experimental data in question indicated that the smooth transition is an inherent property and not merely an artefact of averaging.

8.3 Binaural evaluation

Hitherto the methods for taking unequal hearing into account have usually relied on some arbitrary weighting of 'better' and 'worse' ear, as described in 3.7. For the present Report, a more logically based procedure has been devised. As a practical starting point, equal hearing in both ears is taken as the baseline, and inequalities are handled as degradations from this baseline according to the amount by which the worse ear differs from the better. Better and worse, in this context, refer to the magnitudes of H_{123}. Two main effects result from such degradation, one of which, binaural sensitivity loss, is more readily quantifiable than the other, binaural faculty loss. These effects, though conceptually distinct, coexist and thus jointly affect the resulting disability. Quantitative evidence on binaural faculty loss is comparatively scanty, and for this reason Table A2 has been restricted to the range of interaural HTL differences up to 50 dB.

Binaural sensitivity loss refers to a reduction of perceived loudness, and its magnitude can be calculated from published results relating to the difference of loudness of sounds heard monaurally and binaurally by normal listeners. This loss can be equated to a notional increase in the HTL of the better ear by discounting any contribution by the worse ear. For an interaural HTL difference Δ (worse minus better ear), the effective HTL of the better ear (H_{eff}) is given by

$$H_{eff} = H_{123} + 10 - 33\log(1 + 10^{-\Delta/33}) \qquad \text{Equation 8.3}$$

This expression is equal to H_{123} when $\Delta = 0$ (equal ears) and has a maximum value of 10 dB above H_{123} when the worse ear contributes nothing.

Binaural faculty loss is reflected in impairment of the spatial localization of sounds and decreased binaural ability to resolve spatially distinct dichotic signals; that is, competing sounds such as speech in a noisy background or simultaneous conversations using both ears. Otologically normal persons rarely have ears that are exactly matched, and interaural differences up to 5 dB can be considered normal in respect of these faculties. Above this, the impairments increase gradually with the interaural inequality, but the faculties are not completely extinguished until there is quite a large difference (the value 50 dB is assumed for this Report). The ability to resolve competing sounds also deteriorates with increasing HTL, even with matched ears, particularly in the case of sensorineural hearing loss (SNHL), and this is reflected in the basic relation between HTL and percentage disability in 8.2. However, any additional impairment due to interaural inequality itself diminishes as the overall hearing loss increases, and it is here assumed to do so in proportion to the amount of residual hearing of the better ear (that is, it is proportional to 100% minus the disability percentage for that ear).

The principles outlined above are implemented in Table A2 as augmentations of the percentage disability for a given HTL of the better ear. It was, of course, necessary to this end to quantify the limiting percentage disability corresponding to total loss of hearing in the worse ear, in order to 'calibrate' the sliding scale of augmentations for different degrees of asymmetry. Direct determination of this limiting percentage is, for obvious reasons, impractical, and it has to be derived from common sense and clinical experience. A range of values has been postulated at various times, and for the present Report a value within this range, namely 15%, has been deemed appropriate, of which up to 10% would be accountable to binaural faculty loss.

It should be noted that binaural sensitivity loss is expressed in decibels, and handled as a correction to the HTL of the better ear. By contrast, binaural faculty loss is treated as an adjustment to percentage disability, even though its magnitude depends upon quantities expressed in the decibel domain viz. the HTLs of the two ears. The user of this Report will not have to calculate any corrections for interaural asymmetry explicitly as they are incorporated in Table A2.

8.4 Table of percentage disability

The table of percentage disability is laid out in Table A2 of Annex A in a simple form for use. Each row corresponds to the HTL of the better ear, and each column corresponds to the difference of HTLs between worse and better ear. In order to avoid the awkward fractions ending in 1/3 which would result from averaging HTLs, the rows and columns are labelled instead with the sums and differences of sums of HTLs at the three frequencies. In keeping with the steps of 5 dB recommended for the audiometry, rows and columns are given at intervals of 5 dB. The tabulated values of percentage disability are rounded to the nearest 1%.

The range of HTL is from −10 to +120 dB (−30 to +360 in terms of the sums); interaural HTL differences are given from 0 to 50 dB (0 to 150 in terms of the difference of sums). The disability-rating data on which Table A2 rests do not justify extensions to greater degrees of asymmetry.

An upper limit of 120 dB HL is assumed for a measurement at any frequency. It follows that, for better-ear average HTLs above 70 dB (rows of Table A2 from 215 upwards), the range of interaural difference is restricted by the limit of 120 dB HL attributable to the worse ear. For this reason, there are prohibited areas of Table A2, indicated by blank entries.

Use of Table A2 in practice is described in 9.2.

Summary of chapter recommendations

- The scale relation used to convert impairment to disability follows the sigmoid function shown in Figure 8.1.
- Allowance for loss of binaural sensitivity (Equation 8.3), loss of suprathreshold binaural faculties and the scale relation between impairment and disability are incorporated in Table A2 of Annex A.

Chapter 9
Assessment of disability

9.1 General plan

As the principal objectives and applications of this Report will be for the assessment of disability arising from noise-induced hearing loss (NIHL), this section is written in terms of such assessment. It leaves the reader to adapt the principles and procedures in as appropriate a manner as possible when applying them to disabilities arising from other compensable sensorineural hearing loss or conductive hearing loss.

Figure 9.1 illustrates the sequence of events in the diagnosis of noise-induced hearing loss and its assessment in terms of hearing disability, based on the procedures recommended in this Report. But it could also be used as a framework, or form of check-list, for diagnostic and quantitative assessment of NIHL under any other compensation scheme.

9.1.1 Diagnosis of noise-induced hearing loss

The first requirement in the compensation assessment of a case of alleged NIHL must be that of diagnosis. That is, at least part of the hearing impairment and disability must be diagnosed as having probably been noise-induced. A description of how that diagnosis is made is outside the scope of the present report and the reader should refer to the relevant sections of textbooks (e.g. Alberti, 1987; Hinchcliffe, 1992) and criteria for its diagnosis (Robinson, 1985).

The main inputs to the diagnosis of NIHL are shown in Figure 9.1. Comment will be limited here to those items of importance that seem quite often to be omitted from medicolegal reports on NIHL. These include a note of the claimant's apparent hearing ability while in the clinic, the approximate dates of such relevant events as noticed hearing difficulty, tinnitus and other ear disorders, and experience and duration of post-exposure dullness of hearing and tinnitus. An attempt should be made to quantify the noise exposure in terms of levels of noise, typical daily noise dose, number of days per year of such noise and number of years. This should be adjusted for (estimated) degree and duration of use of earplugs or earmuffs (see Appendix B) and for the protective effect of CHL, according to its degree and how long it is believed or known to have been present, the claimant's medical records (GP, hospital, occupational and military) being potentially helpful in this respect. These noise estimates should

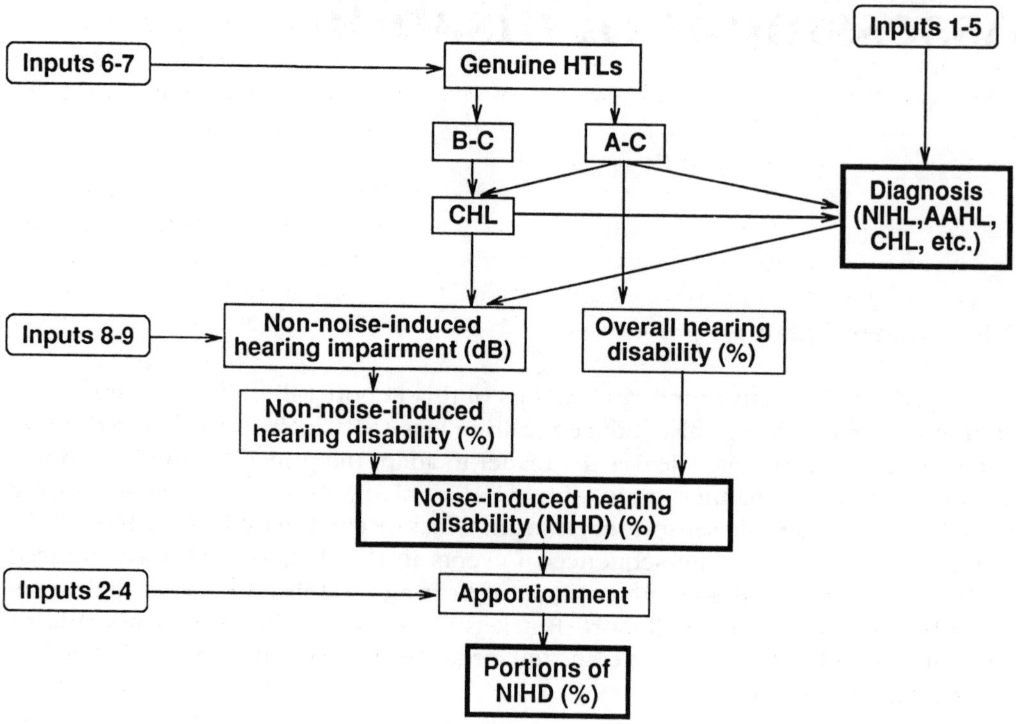

Figure 9.1 Schematic representation of the process of assessment of hearing disability. An example of noise-induced hearing loss is used. Boxes with thick borders represent outcomes of the process.

Key to inputs:

1. Clinical history and examination
2. Noise level data or estimates
3. Noise exposure history, including estimates of daily and yearly exposure, adjusted for use of hearing protection and for any conductive hearing loss (CHL)
4. Medical records
5. Epidemiological data relating hearing loss to noise exposure, sex and age
6. Pure-tone air-conduction and bone-conduction audiometry and other relevant audiological data
7. Indications of spurious hearing threshold levels, and special audiometric tests if needed
8. Notional age-associated hearing loss (AAHL) based on age and sex of claimant
9. Other sensorineural hearing loss (SNHL)

then be used to predict the range of hearing impairments that might arise from such noise exposure, using the published epidemiological and statistical data on the relationships between hearing and noise exposure (Robinson, 1987, 1988a; with some additional guidance from the tables given by Robinson and Shipton, 1977). The hearing impairments actually measured should then be compared with these estimates and with data on the hearing losses to be expected as a function of age alone (BS 6951: 1988; ISO 7029: 1984; data also given in tabular form in Shipton, 1979) in order to assess the probabilities of causation.

The diagnosis of NIHL should not be made unless there is reasonably quantitative information on, or an estimate of, the hazardous noise exposure that is said to have taken place. In the absence of such information, the medical examiner would be well advised to make any diagnosis only provisional; that is, conditional on acoustical confirmation that there had indeed been sufficient noise exposure to have caused the measured hearing impairments.

There are few claimants for compensation for NIHL in whom there is likely to be no element of age-associated hearing loss (AAHL), and a probable element of AAHL therefore needs to be stated as part of the diagnosis. Likewise, there may be contributions to the overall hearing impairment due to other factors, such as CHL, or congenital, infective or traumatic SNHL. These also need to be identified diagnostically as far as possible.

The above has assumed that the genuine hearing threshold levels (GHTL) have been measured. It should be remembered however that in about 20 or 30% of compensation cases there are spurious hearing threshold levels (SHTL). Therefore, before going on to diagnosis and assessment of disability, careful consideration needs to be given to the contents of 6.1 and 6.2 of this Report, covering detection of SHTL and measurement of the GHTL respectively.

9.1.2 Assessment of overall and noise-induced hearing disability

Once the diagnosis of an element of NIHL is established, at least meeting the criterion of 'more probable than not', and the overall hearing impairment measured is believed to be genuine, the overall hearing disability likely to be associated with a typical person having that GHTL can be derived from Table A2.

The attributable disability, in this case the noise-induced hearing disability (NIHD), is obtained by simple subtraction of the constitutional disability, in this case the non-noise-induced hearing disability (NNIHD), from the overall hearing disability (OHD). In most cases the NNIHD is due to nothing more than the presumed component of AAHL. In the absence of any evidence suggesting a greater or lesser than average degree of AAHL, or of other than the average audiometric configuration of AAHL, ISO 7029 data are used to give the notional AAHL for the sex and age of the claimant. The NNIHD is then derived from the notional AAHL based on the relation between disability and H_{123} described in 8.2.

If there are other non-compensable forms of hearing disorder present, in addition to presumed AAHL, the total amount of non-noise-induced hearing impairment (NNIHI) has to be estimated. In the case of CHL this can be quantified within certain limitations and qualifications specified in 7.5; it is then added to the notional AAHL to give the NNIHI (Equation 9.2 in 9.2.3). With additional other cause(s) of SNHL, the case is more complex since different forms of cochlear hearing losses are not arithmetically additive (Robinson, 1991b) and the assessor should use Equation 9.3 or 9.4 in 9.2.3 to calculate how much cochlear hearing impairment would be likely to be present if there had been no noise exposure. To this is added any significant CHL in order to derive the total NNIHL.

9.1.3 *Apportionment*

In many instances there has been only one relevant period of noise exposure, and the NIHD is the final outcome of the assessment that is required. However, in some cases there may have been (i) several different employers, which may include the military, who exposed the claimant to hazardous amounts of noise, (ii) significant leisure noise exposures, (iii) occupational noise exposure prior to the date when knowledge of noise hazards in industry and means of prevention or protection became widely available (in the UK most commonly taken to be 1963), (iv) noise exposure in circumstances of contributory negligence, for example when the claimant unreasonably did not make proper use of earplugs or earmuffs provided for his protection. For all these different periods of exposure, and types of noise including shooting and explosive noises, the total NIHD has to be calculated and then apportioned. The procedures recommended for this are outlined in 10.1.

9.2 How to use the tables

The percentage hearing disability, $D_{overall}$, corresponding to the overall hearing loss, is to be evaluated in all cases by the procedure given in 9.2.1. For cases in which constitutional elements of the hearing loss are involved, the procedure is given in 9.2.2 or 9.2.3.

9.2.1 *General procedure*

Step 1 Combine the two (or more) determinations of the a-c thresholds at 1, 2 and 3 kHz according to the principles in 5.2.3.1 (see also Note 1 below). Sum the resultant HTLs at 1, 2 and 3 kHz for each ear and note the better ear for use with Table A2.

Note 1: where determinations differ by 0 or 5 dB, the better HTL should be taken. Where they differ by 10 dB, the average should be taken.

Step 2 Calculate the difference of the sums (worse ear minus better ear) for use with Table A2.

Note 2: cases in which the difference exceeds 150 may be evaluated by assuming a value of 150, but as such cases tend to be exceptional special considerations may apply.

Step 3 Enter the appropriate row and column of Table A2 and read the percentage disability directly.

9.2.2 *Procedure when there is a single constitutional element*

When there is only one constitutional element, the notional HTLs of each ear that would have existed in the absence of the element attributable to the alleged injury and any other injury of like nature are first determined by the methods given in 7.4 (in the case of AAHL) or 7.5.2 (in the case of CHL). These values are then converted to the notional percentage disability ($D_{constit}$) using the procedure in 9.2.1. The attributable disability is given by:

$$D_{attrib} = D_{overall} - D_{constit} \qquad \text{Equation 9.1}$$

If $D_{constit}$ is greater than $D_{overall}$, the value of D_{attrib} should be taken to be zero.

Note 1: in most cases there will be an element of AAHL. For convenience, Table A3 of Annex A gives disability values directly for males and females between the ages of 18 and 80 years. This table may be used in uncomplicated instances of AAHL instead of using both Table A1 and Table A2.

Note 2: it is possible that $D_{constit}$ may exceed $D_{overall}$ in the case of AAHL, because the notional values of HTL given in Table A1 are derived from median data. In the case of a particular individual, this median value may exceed the whole hearing loss. The apparent paradox arises from the fact that the true threshold shift attributable to AAHL cannot be determined for an individual ear when other hearing losses are overlaid.

Note 3: even where the claimant is young and therefore the notional AAHL is zero, $D_{constit}$ will have a value of 2% (see Table A2).

9.2.3 *Procedure when there is more than one constitutional element*

When there is more than one constitutional element, the combined impairment due to these elements has first to be estimated for each ear. The procedure is then as above. The combined sum of HTLs over the frequencies 1, 2 and 3 kHz (ΣH) due to a conductive component ΣH_C and a sensorineural component ΣH_S (e.g. AAHL) is given by:

$$\Sigma H = \Sigma H_C + \Sigma H_S \qquad \text{Equation 9.2}$$

The sensorineural component may itself be the result of more than one sub-component of SNHL. When there are such multiple sub-components, ΣH_{S1}, ΣH_{S2}, ΣH_{S3} etc., the combined SNHL component is obtained from the following formula:

$$\Sigma H_S = 360[1-(1-\Sigma H_{S1}/360)(1-\Sigma H_{S2}/360)(1-\Sigma H_{S3}/360)...] \qquad \text{Equation 9.3}$$

Note: this is to be applied to the sums of HTLs over the frequencies 1, 2 and 3 kHz and is based on the work of Robinson (1991b).

In the case of two sub-components only (e.g. AAHL and NIHL) this formula reduces to:

$$\Sigma H_S = \Sigma H_{S1} + \Sigma H_{S2} - (\Sigma H_{S1} \times \Sigma H_{S2})/360 \qquad \text{Equation 9.4}$$

Worked examples of the above procedures are given in Appendix A.

Summary of chapter recommendations

- Diagnosis of noise-induced hearing loss should depend on the characteristics of the hearing loss and the impairment expected from the extent of noise exposure, both in relation to age-associated hearing loss.
- Noise-induced hearing disability should be calculated as the difference between the overall hearing disability and the notional hearing disability due to any constitutional hearing loss (Equation 9.1), or due to a combination of constitutional impairments.
- The combination of more than one constitutional element depends on whether they are conductive or sensorineural (Equations 9.2 and 9.3).

Chapter 10
Additional assessment procedures

10.1 Retrospective assessment and rules for apportionment

10.1.1 Derivation of rules for apportionment

In general, assessment of noise-induced hearing disability (NIHD) will be based on current hearing impairment, although in some cases there will be acceptable audiometric data from previous measurements. Lack of previous measurements poses a problem when it is required to apportion NIHD between two (or more) episodes of noise exposure. For example, an individual may have been exposed to noise for two periods of employment with different employers and it is necessary to determine how much of the NIHD is attributable to each employer. In the absence of audiometric measurements obtained before and after each period of noise exposure, apportionment must be based on a theoretical description of how NIHD is expected to accrue under the particular circumstances of exposure. This section describes a method of apportionment based on the theoretical model described by Lutman (1992). It is restricted to exposure to non-impulsive noise. Where there has been exposure to highly impulsive noise (e.g. gunfire), recommendations regarding apportionment are left to the discretion of the medical examiner.

A fundamental assumption of this method is that apportionment is in the domain of disability, rather than in the domain of impairment. The apportionment model makes use of an impairment model proposed by Robinson (1987) to account for the effects of age and noise exposure on hearing threshold levels and extended to multiple episodes of noise exposure by Robinson (1991b). This is transformed to the disability domain using the relationship between disability and impairment proposed by Lutman and Robinson (1992) and also described in Chapter 8 of this Report. Examination of the properties of this disability model by Lutman (1992) indicated that it could be approximated with reasonable accuracy by a simplified relationship of the following form:

$$D \propto \sum_{i=1}^{n} T_i \times (L_i - 84) \qquad \text{Equation 10.1}$$

where D is the total NIHD (current assessment),
T_i is the duration of the ith episode of noise exposure and L_i is the A-weighted

equivalent continuous sound pressure level in decibels of the *i*th episode of noise exposure, integrated over an 8-hour working day ($L_{EP,d}$).

In other words, the total NIHD is proportional to the sum of the products obtained for the component episodes, where each product is obtained by multiplying the duration by the $L_{EP,d}$ minus 84 dB. For example, if a man is exposed to an $L_{EP,d}$ of 90 dB(A) for 10 years, followed by an exposure to an $L_{EP,d}$ of 95 dB(A) for 5 years, the total NIHD is proportional to the sum of (90 – 84) x 10 and (95 – 84) x 5, that is, 60 plus 55. The consequence is that the NIHD should be apportioned in the ratio 60:55. The percentage NIHD to be apportioned is that based on the current assessment.

10.1.2 Method of apportionment

Step 1 For each episode of noise exposure to be considered, it is necessary to determine the duration of the episode and the $L_{EP,d}$. The latter is integrated over the normal working day and applies to jobs where a similar value obtains for each day of the week. Where the daily work schedule varies substantially, a calculation will be required to establish a weekly measure ($L_{EP,w}$). Methods for determining $L_{EP,d}$ and $L_{EP,w}$ values are described in Health and Safety Executive (1989). Where the pattern of working varies from week to week, it will be necessary to split the episode into two or more overlapping components, each with a different noise level, making adjustments to the durations accordingly. For example, if one episode lasted for 5 years and had a cycle of two weeks at 90 dB(A) followed by three weeks at 85 dB(A), this should be considered as an episode lasting two years at 90 dB(A) plus another episode at 85 dB(A) lasting three years.

> Note 1: in determining the value of $L_{EP,d}$ or $L_{EP,w}$ to be used for this purpose, allowance must be made for the regular use of hearing protection. An allowance should be subtracted from $L_{EP,d}$ or $L_{EP,w}$ for the years protected if it is understood that hearing protection was used virtually every time the individual was exposed to hazardous levels of noise: otherwise no allowance should be made. Guidelines on the allowances to be made are given in Appendix B.

Step 2 For each episode of noise exposure the product of the duration in years and the A-weighted equivalent continuous sound pressure level minus 84 dB(A) must be calculated.

> Note 2: for convenience, Table A4 in Appendix A gives this product for levels between 85 and 105 dB(A) and durations between 1 and 45 years. For levels of 84 dB(A) or less, the product is deemed to be zero. Any other combinations must be calculated directly.

Step 3 The NIHD is calculated from the audiometric measurements obtained at the current assessment, as described in Chapter 9 to give a percentage disability value.

Step 4 The percentage disability is divided (apportioned) in the ratio of the products obtained in Step 2 above.

A worked example requiring apportionment is given in Appendix A as Example 10.

10.2 Prognostic assessment

In the years following an assessment, the hearing of an individual can be expected to deteriorate due to ageing, with a consequent increase in hearing disability. However, the NIHD may not increase given that it is defined as the difference between the disability of the exposed individual minus the expected disability for a non-exposed person of the same age and sex (control). The NIHD may either increase or decrease, depending on the relative increases in disability for the exposed individual and the control. This, in turn, depends on (a) the rates of increase in impairment with age in the individual and the control, and also (b) the slope of the disability versus impairment function in the region of interest. Factor (a) is greater for the control (Robinson, 1987), whereas factor (b) is greater for the exposed (more-impaired) individual and thus there is a balance between the two. Lutman (1992) has conducted computer simulations for wide ranges of noise exposure, ages of exposure and ages of assessment and concluded that NIHD may increase with age after the assessment, but that the increase is very slight. It is within the range of variation that could be encompassed by changing the assumptions of the computer model.

For the purposes of this Report, the anticipated increase in NIHD after the date of assessment, sometimes referred to as the prognosis allowance, is deemed to be zero.

10.3 Other considerations

In individual cases, other considerations may have to be taken into account, judged on their own merits. Such considerations may include any tinnitus suffered by the claimant, any vestibular malfunction and the benefit that is to be expected from the use of hearing aids. Prescriptive recommendations to cater for such instances are outside the scope of this Report and no recommendations are given in its main body. However, general guidance is included in Appendix C.

Summary of chapter recommendations

- Apportionment of disability between different episodes of noise exposure should be according to Equation 10.1.
- No allowance should be made for prognosis of noise-induced hearing disability.

Chapter 11
Contents of the medicolegal report

In addition to the patient's name, sex, date of birth, date of examination, present and past medical history (with dates of onset and occurrences) and relevant past history, the report should include a full account of the occupational and/or injury history. The conclusions should cover the following:

Quantitative statements

- *Impairment.* Quantitative statement (or audiogram) of the a-c hearing threshold levels in each ear at 0.25, 0.5, 1, 2, 3, 4, 6 and 8 kHz and of the 1, 2, 3 kHz average. Likewise, a quantitative statement of the b-c thresholds at 1, 2, and 3 kHz where measured, with the 1, 2, 3 kHz b-c averages and average air–bone gaps. A statement is also needed concerning any doubt the tester may have as to the validity of the claimant's responses.
- *Disability.* Quantitative estimates of the overall, constitutional and attributable hearing disability calculated from the above data.
- *Apportionment.* Statement of any information or opinion helpful for apportionment.
- *Quality assurance.* Technical data and quality assurance statements (see 4.4, 4.5 and 5.1.3).

Qualitative statements

- *Diagnosis.* Statement of all factors believed to be substantial contributors to the measured hearing impairment, including an estimation of their relative likelihood and magnitude of effect. Where applicable, the statement should include an estimate of the amount(s) of occupational, leisure and military noise exposure (levels; daily durations, days per year and years; stated dates, extent of usage and type of hearing protection) on which the diagnosis or any apportionment opinion has been based.

  Note 1: diagnoses in most claimants are likely to be multiple, few having no probable element of age-related hearing loss.

  Note 2: SNHL of unknown origin is an acceptable and not uncommon diagnosis.

- *Disability qualifications*. A semi-quantitative opinion is needed on any reasons for regarding the disability to have been under- or over-assessed; for example from evidence of speech audiometric tests and detailed description of hearing difficulties encountered.
- *Handicap*. A semi-quantitative opinion on any factors apparently causing greater or lesser handicap for that particular claimant than is to be expected in the average person with the degree of disability calculated or additionally described above.
- *Tinnitus*. An opinion on the probable cause of the tinnitus. Also a semi-quantitative opinion (see Appendix C) on the 'severity' of any tinnitus. This might be stated on the following descriptive scale:

Trivial – Slight – Moderate – Severe –Very Severe

- *Prognosis*. Opinion on (a) the most likely prognosis of the hearing disorder and/or other relevant symptoms, including tinnitus, and (b) of their possible prognoses, quantifying as far as possible the likelihood and degree of any improvement, deterioration or new development.
- *Treatment*. Opinion on any advisable treatment available from public funds or privately, indicating the probable degrees of amelioration to be expected, their likely costs and relative benefits.
- *Explanations*. Sufficient explanation of the bases of any diagnostic opinion, quantification of impairment, disability or handicap, or any other matter in the report that is not self-evident.
- *Other comments*. Statement of any other factor(s) that may possibly be relevant.

Summary of chapter recommendations

- The medicolegal report should contain all the items listed in this chapter.

Chapter 12
Summary and recommendations

Previous chapters have concluded with short lists of recommendations. In this chapter, those recommendations are brought together, in some instances being combined or expanded. They are arranged according to the following classification: principles and assumptions, main recommendations, general requirements, detailed recommendations, general guidance, implementation. Where appropriate, reference is made to specific sections of the Report.

Principles and assumptions

1. Indirect assessment of disability via a (verifiable) audiometric surrogate is necessary in absence of any satisfactory method of direct assessment.
2. Assessment should focus on the disability expected in the typical (median) person for a given degree of impairment.
3. Preference is given to data on the self-rating of disability in the determination of the relationship between disability and impairment, as opposed to measures based on performance tests.
4. Allowance for age-associated hearing loss should correspond to the impairment expected in the typical (median) person of the same age and sex (notional control subject) as the claimant.
5. In making such allowance, by comparing the claimant with the notional control subject, differences should be computed in the domain of disability. The general principle of assessment of compensable disability is to evaluate the overall disability and then to subtract the disability calculated by omitting the attributable component of the hearing loss. This subtraction is expressed in Equation 9.1.

Main recommendations

6. The audiometric surrogate for disability should be the average of the pure-tone thresholds at the frequencies 1, 2 and 3 kHz.
7. The scale relation between disability and hearing threshold level that should be used is curvilinear over the whole range and derived from experimental data. The recommended relationship is illustrated in Figure 8.1 and is embodied in Table A2 of Annex A.

8. A concrete proposal is made concerning disability when the sensitivity of the ears is unequal. This involves adjustment for the loss of binaural sensitivity and also the loss of supra-threshold binaural faculties which assist in localization and processing signals in noise. The adjustment for loss of binaural sensitivity is given by Equation 8.3. This, and also adjustment for loss of supra-threshold binaural faculties, is embodied in Table A2 of Annex A.
9. Allowance for age-associated hearing loss should be according to ISO 7029.
10. The notional disability due to constitutional components is obtained by converting the notional hearing threshold level due to those components into disability.
11. In calculating notional constitutional hearing loss, the rule for combination of more than one element depends on whether they are conductive or sensorineural. Specific rules for combination are given by Equations 9.2 and 9.3.
12. Estimation of conductive hearing loss from measurement of the air–bone gap should take account of the possibility of positive air–bone gaps arising out of biological variation and measurement uncertainty. A specific rule for determining the conductive hearing loss to be used in assessment calculations is given in Table 7.1.
13. Apportionment of disability between different episodes of noise exposure, should be based on the noise levels and durations of the exposures and whether hearing protection was worn during each exposure. A specific rule for apportionment calculations is given by Equation 10.1.
14. No allowance should be made for prognosis of noise-induced hearing disability.

General requirements

15. Basic audiometric testing and reporting of results should follow the methods recommended by the British Society of Audiology.
16. Testing should be carried out by an appropriately qualified person, as defined in 5.3.
17. It is the responsibility of the medical examiner to ensure appropriate quality assurance, including adequate audiometer calibration.

Detailed recommendations

18. Equipment for audiometry should comply with BS 5966 with a direct link to national standards for hearing levels.
19. The use of noise-excluding earphone enclosures is not recommended.
20. Background noise levels for audiometry should preferably meet the requirements of BS 6655, but will be acceptable for measurements at 1, 2 and 3 kHz if they meet the relaxed requirements given in Table 4.1.
21. Two separate determinations should be made of each of the air-conduction thresholds at 1, 2 and 3 kHz for each ear.
22. When there is any indication of spurious hearing threshold levels, as defined in 6.1, cortical electric response audiometry should be applied and interpreted as described in 6.2.

General guidance

23. Diagnosis of noise-induced hearing loss should depend on the characteristics of the hearing loss and the hearing loss expected from the extent of noise exposure, both in relation to the expected age-associated hearing loss.
24. The medicolegal report should contain all the items listed in Chapter 11.

Implementation

25. The Working Group recommends that this Report be regarded as superseding the recommendations of the former working group that reported in 1983.

List of symbols and abbreviations

AAHL	age-associated hearing loss
AAOO	American Academy of Ophthalmology and Otolaryngology
AATS	age-associated threshold shift
ABG	air–bone gap
ABR	auditory brainstem response
a-c	air conduction
ACAE	Advisory Committee on Audiological Equipment (DHSS)
AMA	American Medical Association
ART	acoustic reflex threshold*
BAAP	British Association of Audiological Physicians
BAOL	British Association of Otolaryngologists
b-c	bone conduction
BS	British Standard (of the British Standards Institution)
BSA	British Society of Audiology
CERA	cortical electric response audiometry
CHABA	Committee on Hearing Bioacoustics and Biomechanics (of the US National Academy of Science)
CHL	conductive hearing loss
D	percentage disability (with subscripts denoting its attribution)
dB	decibel, unit of level
dB(A)	unit of A-weighted sound pressure level
DHSS	Department of Health and Social Security, UK*
DSS	Department of Social Security, UK
f	frequency (of pure tone)*
GHTL	genuine hearing threshold level

* Found only in the Glossary.

H	hearing threshold level (with subscript denoting relevant audiometric frequencies or ascribing the HTL to a disorder)
HL	hearing level in dB (produced by an audiometer)
HMS	Hearing Measurement Scale (W.G. Noble)
HPL	half-peak level (in speech audiometry)*
HPLE	half-peak level elevation (in speech audiometry)*
HTL	hearing threshold level (of an ear)
Hz	hertz, unit of frequency
IEC	International Electrotechnical Commission (also prefix to Standards issued by IEC)
ISO	International Organization for Standardization (also prefix to Standards issued by ISO)
kHz	kilohertz
L	sound pressure level
$L_{EP,d}$	daily noise exposure level. Also $L_{EP,w}$ – weekly
mm^2	square millimetres
MRC	Medical Research Council, UK
N	newton, unit of force
NAMAS	National Measurement Accreditation Service, UK
NEH	noise exposure history
NIHD	noise-induced hearing disability
NIHL	noise-induced hearing loss
NIPTS	noise-induced permanent threshold shift*
NLDE	noise level data/estimates
NNIHD	non-noise-induced hearing disability
NPL	National Physical Laboratory, UK
NSH	National Study of Hearing (conducted by MRC Institute of Hearing Research)
ODS	optimum discrimination score*
OHD	overall hearing disability
PTS	permanent threshold shift*
RETFL	reference equivalent threshold (vibratory) force level*
RETSPL	reference equivalent threshold sound pressure level*
RSRTL	reference speech recognition threshold level*
SFSRA	sweep-frequency self-recording audiometry (or audiometer)
SHL	speech hearing level*
SHTL	spurious hearing threshold level
SL	sensation level*

SLM	sound level meter*
SNHL	sensorineural hearing loss
SPL	sound pressure level*
SRT	speech reception level*
SRTL	speech recognition threshold level*
T	duration of noise exposure
TTS	temporary threshold shift*
U	parameter used in the formula for *D*
WHO	World Health Organization
Δ	interaural HTL difference
µN	micronewton
µPa	micropascal
Σ*H*	sum of HTLs at 1, 2 and 3 kHz

Glossary

The definitions below are taken mainly from ISO, IEC and WHO, adapted where necessary.

air conduction (a-c)
The transmission of sound through the outer and middle ear to the internal ear.

acoustic admittance
Reciprocal of *acoustic impedance*.

acoustic coupler
A cavity of specified shape and volume which is used for the calibration of an earphone in conjunction with a calibrated microphone to measure the sound pressure developed within the cavity. A simplified type of *artificial ear*.

acoustic impedance
Quotient of a sound pressure by the volume velocity produced by it.

acoustic reflex
Contraction of the stapedius muscle in response to an auditory eliciting stimulus.

acoustic reflex threshold (ART)
The least sound pressure level of a sound that elicits the acoustic reflex.

admittance (aural)
See *immittance*.

age–associated hearing loss (AAHL)
Term used to describe hearing loss primarily related to age but which may include components with unidentified aetiology. See *presbyacusis*.

air–bone gap (ABG)
Of an ear, hearing threshold level by air conduction minus hearing threshold level by bone conduction.

apportionment
The division of one or more measures of malfunction of the auditory system, or their effects, into components attributable to various causes according to their relative contributions (known, inferred, or estimated). In its quantitative connotation, apportionment is applied to percentage disability or, for some purposes, to threshold shifts in decibels.

articulation function
See *speech recognition curve* (synonymous).

artificial ear
A device for the calibration of an earphone which presents to the earphone an acoustic impedance equivalent to the impedance presented by the average human ear. It is equipped with a calibrated microphone for the measurement of the sound pressure developed by the earphone. See *ear simulator*; *acoustic coupler*.

artificial mastoid
A device used to load a bone vibrator, dynamically and statically, enabling the bone vibrator to be calibrated. The device includes a mechano-electric transducer (usually piezoelectric). The mechanical impedance of the device is made to simulate that presented to a vibrator when placed over the average human mastoid process. Used to calibrate bone-conduction audiometers and to test bone-conduction hearing aids. See *mechanical coupler*.

audiogram
Pure-tone audiogram: a chart or table of a person's hearing threshold levels for pure tones at different frequencies. See also *speech audiogram*.

audiometer
Pure-tone audiometer: an electroacoustical instrument, equipped (for air conduction) with two earphones and headset, which provides pure tones of specified frequencies at known sound pressure levels, used to determine hearing threshold levels, one ear at a time. For bone conduction the audiometer is also equipped with a bone vibrator. For clinical use, both facilities are required, as well as means of generating calibrated masking noise; an input port is also usually provided for connection to an external signal source.

A *manual audiometer* is one in which the signal presentations, frequency and hearing level selection, and the noting of the subject's responses, are performed manually.

A *self-recording audiometer* (also known as an *automatic-recording audiometer*) is one in which the frequency selection or variation and the recording of the subject's responses are implemented automatically, and in which the level increases or decreases continuously with the direction of change under the subject's control. A self-recording audiometer may have facilities for presenting fixed frequencies or a continuously variable (sweep) frequency, or both; it may also provide both continuous and pulsed tone outputs (see *Békésy audiometry*).

A *computer-controlled audiometer* is one in which the control functions, and often the calculation and display of hearing threshold levels derived from the subject's responses, are implemented by a computer.

A *speech audiometer* is an instrument for the measurement of hearing using speech test material. A pure-tone audiometer is often adaptable to a speech audiometer by using the external input port.

audiometric zero
See *reference zero* (synonymous).

audiometry
Measurement of auditory function.

Pure-tone audiometry usually means the determination of a person's hearing threshold levels for pure tones by air conduction under monaural earphone listening conditions, or by bone conduction. See also *Békésy audiometry; immittance audiometry; speech audiometry*.

A-weighted sound pressure level
The sound pressure level of a signal which has been passed through an 'A' filter whereby both low- and high-frequency components are attenuated without affecting the components near 1000 Hz. The unit is the decibel but it is usual to distinguish between this and other uses of the decibel by writing the unit as dB(A). See *frequency weighting*.

bandwidth
The difference between the upper and lower limits of a frequency band. Bandwidth may be expressed in hertz (Hz) or as a fraction of an octave centred on the mid-frequency of the band (usually the geometric centre frequency).

Békésy audiometry
A form of self-recording pure-tone audiometry in which diagnostic use can be made of differences between the thresholds obtained using pulsed and continuous tone presentations. It is recommended to reserve this term for audiometry using a continuous frequency sweep (glide tone) to distinguish it from self-recording audiometry using fixed frequencies.

binaural squelch
The effective increase in signal-to-noise ratio conferred by binaural hearing when the signal and noise sources are at different angles of incidence. The binaural squelch effect arises out of cues available from differences in intensity and time-of-arrival of the signals at the two ears.

bone conduction (b-c)
The transmission of sound to the internal ear primarily by means of mechanical vibration of the cranial bones.

bone vibrator
An electromechanical transducer designed to produce the sensation of hearing by vibrating the cranial bones.

compliance
See *immittance*.

conductive hearing loss (CHL)
Hearing loss caused by blockage of the outer ear or by derangement of the middle ear, resulting in a reduction of sound energy reaching the internal ear.

coupler
See *acoustic coupler; mechanical coupler*.

decibel (dB)
The unit for measuring the relative magnitude of a quantity based on a logarithmic scale. See *sound pressure level; A-weighted sound pressure level; hearing level; hearing threshold level*.

disability
In the general context of health experience, a disability is defined by WHO as any restriction or lack (resulting from an impairment) of ability to perform an activity in the manner or within the range considered normal for a human being. Disability represents disturbances at the level of the *person* and which express themselves in everyday life.

discrimination score
See *speech recognition score* (synonymous).

earmuff
A hearing protector designed to enclose the pinna.

earphone
An electroacoustic transducer operating from an electrical system to an acoustic system and designed to be applied to the ear, usually without leakage. See *headphones*.

earplug
A hearing protector which is inserted into the ear canal.

ear protector
See *hearing protector*.

ear simulator
Synonymous with *artificial ear*, but now the preferred term.

filter
A device which modifies the frequency spectrum of a signal, usually while it is in electrical form.

frequency
The rate of vibration of air particles which constitutes a sound. The unit is the hertz (Hz) equal to one cycle per second.

frequency band
A frequency interval which has an upper and lower limit and includes all the frequencies within this range. See *bandwidth*.

frequency weighting
Modification of the frequency spectrum of a signal by means of a filter having one of the standardized response characteristics known as 'A', 'B', 'C' etc. The 'A' weighting is the most commonly used.

half optimum speech recognition level
For a given listener with an *optimum speech recognition score* of less than 100%, for a specified speech signal and a specified manner of signal presentation, the *speech level* at which half of the *optimum speech recognition score* is obtained and which is lower than the *optimum speech level*. See *speech level; optimum speech level; optimum speech recognition score*.

half-peak level (HPL)
See *half optimum speech recognition level* (synonymous).

half-peak level elevation (HPLE)
Of a given ear, the difference between *half optimum speech recognition level* and the *reference speech recognition threshold level*.

handicap
In the general context of health experience, a handicap is defined by WHO as a disadvantage for a given individual, resulting from an impairment or a disability, that limits or prevents the fulfilment of a role that is normal (depending on age, sex and social and cultural factors) for that individual.

head shadow
The difference in sound levels arriving at the two ears when the direction of incident sound is at an angle to the median plane. The effect of head shadow is greater at high frequencies than low frequencies.

headphones
An assembly comprising two earphones and a headband or equivalent device to hold these in place with a specified force.

hearing level (HL)
For a pure tone, at a specified frequency, type of transducer and manner of application, the *sound pressure level* (or the *vibratory force level*) of a pure tone, produced by the transducer in a specified artificial ear or acoustic coupler (or mechanical coupler) minus the appropriate *reference equivalent threshold sound pressure level* (or

reference equivalent threshold force level). For a correctly calibrated audiometer it is equal to the dial setting.

hearing level for speech
See *speech hearing level* (synonymous).

hearing loss
The amount by which an individual's hearing threshold level changes for the worse as a result of some adverse influence, expressed in decibels. Also used loosely to mean a symptom of hearing disorder, and also (but incorrectly) as a synonym for *hearing threshold level*. Note that a person whose hearing has changed from –15 to –5 dB hearing threshold level has suffered a loss, but a person who started with and still has a hearing threshold level of +5 dB (or for that matter +15 dB) has lost nothing. The term *hearing loss* is also used in conjunction with descriptors, e.g. *age-associated, noise-induced, conductive, sensorineural etc.*

hearing protector
A general term embracing earmuff, earplug and helmet (or other noise-excluding device) worn on the head or in the ear canal.

hearing threshold level (HTL)
Of a given ear, for a specified frequency and type of transducer, the threshold of hearing at that frequency, expressed as *hearing level*. Note that *hearing threshold level* is a property of the ear under test whereas *hearing level* refers only to the sound (or vibration) generated by a measuring instrument.

hertz (Hz)
The unit of frequency (see *frequency*).

immittance (aural)
A generic term embracing acoustic impedance, acoustic admittance, acoustic compliance, equivalent air volume, and related quantities determined by *immittance audiometry*.

immittance audiometry
Determination of the acoustic properties (impedance, admittance etc.) of the middle ear. See *tympanometry; acoustic reflex threshold*.

impairment
In the general context of health experience, an impairment is defined by WHO as any loss or abnormality of psychological, physiological, or anatomical structure or function. Impairments represent disturbances at the level of the *organ*.

impedance (acoustic)
See *immittance*.

masking

1. The process by which the threshold of hearing of one sound is raised due to the presence of another sound (the 'masker'), usually noise.
2. The amount by which the *hearing threshold level* (or *speech recognition threshold level*) of a given ear is so raised (masking threshold shift), expressed in decibels.

Ipsilateral masking refers to the masking of a signal by a noise delivered to the same ear as the signal.

Contralateral masking occurs where the noise has its masking effect on a signal reaching the non-test (contralateral) ear.

Cross-masking occurs where the noise, delivered contralaterally, crosses the head and then reaches the test ear, so masking the signal in the test ear.

Central masking refers to the case where noise causes a threshold elevation in the absence of, or additional to, any ipsilateral, contralateral or cross-masking effect; it is due to interactions within the central nervous system between the separate neural inputs derived from the signal and the noise.

mechanical coupler

A device designed to present a specified mechanical impedance to a vibrator applied with a specified static force and equipped with a mechano-electrical transducer to measure the vibratory force level at the surface of contact between vibrator and mechanical coupler. A simplifed kind of *artificial mastoid*.

mechanical impedance

Quotient of a vibratory force by the vibratory velocity it produces.

noise

1. In general, any sound which is undesired by the recipient. In the context of assessing hearing damage any audible extraneous sound should be regarded as noise.
2. A class of sound, derived from an electrical signal and used for specific test purposes, e.g. in audiology, characterized by having a continuous spectrum over a defined frequency band.

Wideband noise consists of a wide range of audio frequencies.

Narrow band noise (e.g. one-third-octave band noise) consists of all frequencies within the band and negligible power outside the band.

White noise has equal power per unit bandwidth over a specified frequency range.

Pink noise has equal power in equal percentage bandwidths (i.e. in bands f_1 to f_2 where f_1/f_2 is constant), over a specified frequency range.

Random noise is a signal whose instantaneous value varies randomly with time.

noise-excluding headset
A headphone set in which each earphone is surrounded by an earcup to provide additional attenuation of ambient noise.

occluded ear simulator
A device simulating the acoustic properties of the tympanic membrane and its attached structures.

occlusion effect
Generally applied to the change (usually an increase) in level of a bone-conducted signal reaching the internal ear when an earphone or an earplug is placed over or at the entrance of the ear canal, thereby forming an enclosed air volume in the external ear. The effect is greatest at low frequencies.

octave
A frequency ratio of 2 to 1. An octave band has a bandwidth one octave wide. The sound pressure level of a sound which has been passed through an octave band pass filter is termed the *octave band sound pressure level*. Similarly for *one-third octave bands*, there being three such bands in each octave band, the frequency ratio of the band limits in each one-third octave band being 1.259 (cube root of 2).

optimum discrimination score (ODS)
See *optimum speech recognition score* (synonymous).

optimum speech level
For a given listener, a specified speech signal and a specified manner of signal presentation, the *speech level* at which maximum *speech recognition score* occurs.

optimum speech recognition score
For a given listener, a specified speech signal and a specified manner of signal presentation, the *speech recognition score* obtained at the *optimum speech level*.

permanent threshold shift
The component of threshold shift which shows no recovery with the passage of time when the apparent cause has been removed. *Noise-induced permanent threshold shift* (NIPTS) is the component of PTS specifically attributable to noise exposure. The PTS may also include an *age-associated hearing loss* (AAHL), a pathological component, or both.

presbyacusis
Hearing disorder which accompanies ageing in the absence of other identifiable causes, and which is causing hearing difficulties in an older person. This term should not be confused with *age-associated hearing loss*.

pure tone
A sound having a single frequency and whose sound pressure varies sinusoidally with time.

recruitment (of loudness)
A manifestation of auditory dysfunction which is characterized by a raised threshold and by a more rapid rate of increase of loudness with sensation level than for a normal ear.

reference equivalent threshold force level (RETFL)
See *reference zero*.

reference equivalent threshold sound pressure level (RETSPL)
See *reference zero*.

reference speech recognition curve
For a specified speech signal and a specified manner of presentation, a curve that describes the median *speech recognition score* as a function of *speech level* for a sufficiently large number of otologically normal test persons of both sexes, aged between 18 and 30 years inclusive and for whom the test material is appropriate.

reference speech recognition threshold level (RSRTL)
For a specified speech signal and a specified manner of presentation, the mean value of the *speech recognition threshold levels* of a sufficiently large number of otologically normal test persons of both sexes, aged between 18 and 30 years inclusive and for whom the test material is appropriate.

reference zero
For *pure-tone air-conduction audiometry* a set of sound pressure levels of pure tones at audiometric frequencies, which corresponds to the normal threshold of hearing of young persons. For each frequency the value is expressed by the sound pressure level measured in an acoustic coupler or artificial ear when the earphone, driven by a specific electrical signal, is placed on the coupler. This value is known as the *reference equivalent threshold sound pressure level* (RETSPL) for the frequency in question. The specific electrical signal is such that the sound pressure level it generates under the earphone when placed on the average human ear corresponds to the modal value of the thresholds of hearing of a group of otologically normal persons aged between 18 and 30 years. The values of RETSPL for a range of commonly used earphones are given in BS 2497 Parts 5 and 6 and in ISO 389:1991.

For *pure-tone bone-conduction audiometry*, the reference zero is defined analogously by *reference equivalent threshold (vibratory) force level* (RETFL) when the bone vibrator is loaded by a specified mechanical coupler. The RETFL values are specified in BS 6950 (identical to ISO 7566). Use of acceleration level for the reference zero is obsolete.

sensation level (SL)
For a given ear, the level of a sound above the threshold of hearing for the same sound, expressed in decibels.

sensorineural hearing loss (SNHL)
A hearing loss due to a lesion or disorder of the internal ear or of the auditory nervous system.

sound level meter (SLM)
An instrument designed to measure a frequency- and time-weighted value of the sound pressure level. It consists of a microphone, amplifier, square-law rectifier, averaging circuits, and indicating instrument, having a specified performance in respect of directivity, frequency response, rectification characteristic, and time-weighted averaging. The instrument is normally equipped with the 'F' and 'S' time-weightings, and possibly also with the 'I' time-weighting as an aid to measuring fluctuating sounds. With suitable circuitry it can also perform frequency analyses, usually in one-octave or one-third-octave bands.

sound pressure level (SPL)
The sound pressure level of a sound in decibels, is equal to 20 times the logarithm to the base 10 of the ratio of the root mean square sound pressure to the reference sound pressure 20 μPa (2×10^{-5} Pa).

speech audiogram
For an individual, a chart or graph depicting the *speech recognition curve* for that person. It may also indicate the person's *speech detection threshold*.

speech audiometry
The presentation of speech material (usually word lists) to determine the percentage of material correctly detected or correctly identified. In the simplest form, listening is monaural by earphone in quiet to recorded material. Variations include live-voice presentation, free-field binaural listening, added noise etc. Results are displayed on a *speech audiogram*.

speech detection threshold level
For a given listener, a specified speech signal and a specified manner of presentation, the speech level of the test material at which it is detected (but not necessarily understood) in a specified percentage of the trials, usually 50%.

speech hearing level (SHL)
For a specified speech signal and a specified manner of signal presentation, the *speech level* minus the appropriate *reference speech recognition threshold level*.

speech level
The sound pressure level (or vibratory force level) of a speech signal as measured in an appropriate acoustic coupler, artificial ear or sound field (or on a mechanical coupler) with specified frequency weighting and time weighting. For single test items, the maximum measured sound pressure level or vibratory force level is used; for sentences and running speech, the average of the maximum values for each scored word is used. An ISO committee draft (ISO/CD 8253-3) recommends use of the 'C' frequency weighting and the 'I' time weighting.

speech reception threshold (SRT)
See *speech recognition threshold level* (synonymous)

speech recognition curve
For a given listener, a specified speech signal and a specified manner of signal presentation, a curve which describes that person's *speech recognition score* as a function of *speech level.*

speech recognition score
For a given listener, a specified speech signal and specified manner of presentation, and at a *specified speech* level, the percentage of test items correctly identified. The method of scoring will influence the result and should therefore also be specified.

speech recognition threshold level (SRTL)
For a given listener, a specified speech signal and a specified manner of signal presentation, the speech level at which a specified percentage (usually 50%) of the test items can be correctly identified by that person.

temporary threshold shift (TTS)
The component of threshold shift which shows recovery with the passage of time after the apparent cause has been removed.

threshold of hearing
The minimum level of a sound which is just audible in given conditions on a specified fraction of trials (conventionally 50%). In quiet conditions this is referred to as the *absolute threshold*. In the presence of a masking sound or noise it is called the *masked threshold*.

threshold shift
The difference, in decibels, between the hearing threshold levels of a person measured on two separate occasions. If the threshold shift progressively diminishes with passage of time when the cause (usually noise) has ceased, it is referred to as *temporary threshold shift* (TTS), otherwise as *permanent threshold shift* (PTS).

time weighting
The characteristic of the averaging process which is applied to the square-law rectified electrical signal in a sound level meter. The 'S' and 'F' time weightings provide smoothing over periods of the order 2 s and 250 ms respectively and yield the same result for steady sounds, but not for time-varying sounds, e.g. vehicle noise or speech. The 'I' weighting has a fast rise time, slow decay time, characteristic, sometimes used to measure impulsive sound. 'Peak' weighting gives a measure of the maximum instantaneous sound pressure in a sound waveform.

tinnitus
A sensation of sound which does not have an external acoustic or mechanical stimulus and has no manifest physiological origin. Occasionally tinnitus is associated with an externally detectable component, sometimes called *objective tinnitus*.

Tullio phenomenon
Vestibular disturbance induced by a concurrent acoustic stimulus.

tympanometry
Determination of the acoustic immittance of an ear as a function of the difference between the air pressure applied to the external ear canal and the ambient atmospheric pressure. The result is displayed graphically as a *tympanogram*.

Appendix A
Worked examples

The following are examples of assessment of compensable disability, for various combinations of age, sex, noise-induced hearing loss and conductive or other defect. Pure-tone hearing threshold levels (HTL) are expressed as sets of three numbers representing the thresholds at the frequencies 1, 2 and 3 kHz rounded to the nearest 5 dB unless stated otherwise. However, for simplicity, air–bone gaps are expressed as the average across those three frequencies. Most examples require the HTLs at the three frequencies to be added together, and for convenience this sum is also given in the preamble (using the Σ notation to indicate summation). An exception to the above is Example 2 where the HTLs have been measured to the nearest 1 dB.

Examples 1 and 2 are concerned with summing HTLs across the three frequencies and with obtaining the definitive HTL from the two replicate measures. Examples 3–9 each follow a similar pattern and are laid out to emphasize this pattern. Two percentage disability values are calculated: one for the *claimant* as seen at assessment and one for the notional *control*. The notional control has hearing thresholds expected for a person of the same age and sex, and any other constitutional impairments found in the claimant, but without the attributable impairment. The difference between these two disability values is then calculated, giving the attributable disability. Example 10 demonstrates the calculation of apportionment between several periods of noise exposure.

Example 1

Determine for each ear the definitive genuine hearing threshold level (GHTL) summed over the frequencies 1, 2 and 3 kHz (ΣH), where the individual GHTLs measured were slightly different between test and re-test, as follows. In the left ear: first test 35, 45 and 75 dB at 1, 2 and 3 kHz respectively; second test 40, 50, 65 dB. In the right ear: first test 35, 45, and 65 dB at 1, 2 and 3 kHz respectively; second test 45, 45 and 70 dB.

Method. Apply the procedures in 5.2.3.1 and 9.2.1, Step 1 and Note 1. Where the difference between the two threshold determinations is 5 dB take the lower (more acute) threshold; where it is 10 dB take the average.

	1	2	3 kHz	
Left ear:				
Test 1:	35	45	75	
Test 2:	40	50	65	
Value to be taken:	35	45	70	
Sum (Σ*H*):				150 dB
Right ear:				
Test 1:	35	45	65	
Test 2:	45	45	70	
Value to be taken:	40	45	65	
Sum (Σ*H*):				150 dB

The result is 150 dB for each ear. Hence the better-ear value is 150 dB and the difference between ears is 0 dB. These values are required to enter Table A2 to obtain the deemed hearing disability.

Example 2

Determine the definitive genuine hearing threshold level (GHTL) summed over the frequencies 1, 2 and 3 kHz (ΣH), where the individual GHTLs were measured to the nearest 1 dB by fixed-frequency self-recording audiometry and were slightly different between test and re-test. Do this for the left ear only. The thresholds obtained from the self-recorded audiogram for that ear were as follows: first test 24, 26, 43 dB at 1, 2 and 3 kHz respectively; second test 22, 24 and 51 dB.

Method. Applying the procedure in 5.2.2, adjust the values obtained by self-recording audiometry to be equivalent to those for manual audiometry, and round to the nearest 5 dB. Then follow the procedure in Example 1 to obtain Σ*H*.

		1	2	3 kHz	
Test 1:					
	Raw measurement:	24	26	43	
	Adjust for self-recording:	27	29	46	
	Round to nearest 5 dB:	25	30	45	
Test 2:					
	Raw measurement:	22	24	51	
	Adjust for self-recording:	25	27	54	
	Round to nearest 5 dB:	25	25	55	
Value to be taken:		25	25	50	
Sum (Σ*H*):					100 dB

In Example 3 and subsequent examples, the principle embodied in Equation 9.1 has been used. But in these particular cases, the attributable disability (D_{attrib}) is identified by a particular cause and is termed noise-induced hearing disability (NIHD). Likewise, the constitutional disability ($D_{constit}$) is non-noise-induced disability (NNIHD).

Example 3

Find the noise-induced hearing disability (NIHD) of a man aged 60, with NIHL and presumed age-associated hearing loss (AAHL) only. Genuine hearing threshold levels (GHTL) are 30,45,75 dB (Σ=150) in both ears.

Method. NIHD is the difference between overall hearing disability (OHD) and non-noise-induced hearing disability (NNIHD), in this case due solely to presumed AAHL:

Claimant:	Sum the GHTL to give Σ*H* values			(Better ear 150, difference 0)
	OHD	=	38%	(Table A2)
Control:	NNIHD	=	7%	(Table A3)
Difference:	NIHD	=	38% – 7%	
	Result	=	31%	

Example 4

Find the noise-induced hearing disability (NIHD) of a man aged 23 with NIHL and presumed AAHL only. Genuine hearing threshold levels (GHTL) are 0,10,20 dB (Σ=30) in both ears.

Method. NIHD is the difference between overall hearing disability (OHD) and non-noise-induced hearing disability (NNIHD), in this case due solely to presumed AAHL:

Claimant:	Sum the GHTL to give Σ*H* values			(Better ear 30, difference 0)
	OHD	=	6%	(Table A2)
Control:	NNIHD	=	2%	(Table A3)
Difference:	NIHD	=	6% – 2%	
	Result	=	4%	

Note: although the notional AAHL is zero (see Table A1), there is still a 2% correction to be made (see Table A2).

Example 5

Find the noise-induced hearing disability (NIHD) of a woman aged 60 with NIHL and presumed AAHL only. Genuine hearing threshold levels (GHTL) are 0,5,15 dB (Σ=20) in both ears.

Method. NIHD is the difference between overall hearing disability (OHD) and non-noise-induced hearing disability (NNIHD), in this case due solely to presumed AAHL.

Claimant:	Sum the GHTL to give ΣH values		(Better ear 20, difference 0)
	OHD	= 4%	(Table A2)
Control:	NNIHD	= 6%	(Table A3)
Difference:	NIHD	= 4% – 6%	
	Result	= –2% (to be regarded as 0%)	

Note: there is no greater overall hearing disability than is to be expected from AAHL alone in the median woman of her age.

Example 6

Find the noise-induced hearing disability (NIHD) of a man aged 70, with NIHL, presumed AAHL and a middle-ear disorder. Genuine hearing threshold levels (GHTL) are 50,70,90 dB (Σ=210) in both ears, average air–bone gap is 20 dB in both ears (and there is no reason to suspect a secondary sensorineural hearing loss).

Method. The NIHD is the difference between the overall hearing disability (OHD) and the non-noise-induced hearing disability (NNIHD), in this case due to the combined hearing threshold level components of presumed AAHL and the conductive hearing loss (CHL) due to middle-ear disorder:

Claimant:	Sum the GHTL to give ΣH values				(Better ear 210, difference 0)
	OHD	=		62%	(Table A2)
Control:	ΣAAHL	=	60 dB		(Table A1)
	ΣCHL	=	30 dB		(6 X (ABG – 15 dB); see 7.5.2)
	Σ(AAHL+CHL)	=	90 dB		
	NNIHD	=		18%	(Table A2; better ear 90, difference 0)
Difference:	NIHD	=		62% – 18%	
	Result	=		44%	

Example 7

Find the noise-induced hearing disability (NIHD) of a man aged 58, with NIHL, presumed AAHL and a known pre-exposure sensorineural hearing loss (other SNHL) of non-progressive type. Genuine hearing threshold levels (GHTL) are 30,45,45 dB (Σ=120) in both ears; other SNHL is 15,20,25 dB (Σ=60) in both ears.

Method. The NIHD is the difference between the overall hearing disability (OHD) and the non-noise-induced hearing disability (NNIHD), in this case due to the combined hearing threshold level components of presumed AAHL and the other SNHL.

Claimant:	Sum the GHTL to give Σ*H* values			(Better ear 120, difference 0)
	OHD	=	27%	(Table A2)
Control:	ΣAAHL	=	35 dB	(Table A1)
	Σ(other SNHL)	=	60 dB	(measured pre-exposure)
	Σ(combined AAHL and other SNHL)			(Equation 9.4)
		=	35+60 – (35 x 60/360) dB	
		=	95 – 6 dB	
		=	90 dB	(to nearest 5 dB)
	NNIHD	=	18%	(Table A2; better-ear 90, difference 0)
Difference:	NIHD	=	OHD – (NNIHD for notional AAHL + other SNHL)	
		=	27%–18%	
	Result	=	9%	

Example 8

Find the noise-induced hearing disability (NIHD) of a man aged 48 with NIHL and presumed AAHL only. Genuine hearing threshold levels (GHTL) are 35,45,55 dB (Σ=135) on the left side and 25,30,45 dB (Σ=100) on the right side.

Method. NIHD is the difference between overall hearing disability and non-noise-induced hearing disability (NNIHD), in this case solely due to presumed AAHL.

Claimant:	Sum the GHTL to give Σ*H* values			(Better ear 100, difference 35)
	OHD	=	26%	(Table A2)
Control:	NNIHD	=	4%	(Table A3)
Difference:	NIHD	=	26% – 4%	
	Result	=	22%	

Example 9

Find the noise-induced hearing disability (NIHD) of a woman aged 68 with NIHL in both ears, presumed AAHL, and in the left ear only a middle-ear disorder probably due to otosclerosis and present for about 20 years. Genuine hearing threshold levels (GHTL) are 50, 65, 75 dB (Σ=190) on the left side and 30, 45, 60 dB (Σ=135) on the right; the average air–bone gap (ABG) is 21.7 dB on the left (and there is no reason to suspect a secondary sensorineural hearing loss).

Method. The NIHD is the difference between the overall hearing disability (OHD) and the non-noise-induced hearing disability (NNIHD), in this case due to the non-noise-induced hearing loss (NNIHL), comprising presumed AAHL only in the right ear and presumed AAHL plus conductive hearing loss (CHL) in the left ear.

Claimant:	Sum the GHTL to give ΣH values				(Better ear 135, difference 55)
	OHD	=		41%	(Table A2)
Control:	ΣAAHL	=	45 dB		(Table A1)
	ΣNNIHL (right)	=	45 dB		(AAHL only)
	ΣCHL (left)	=	40 dB		(6 x (ABG – 15 dB); see 7.5.2)
	ΣNNIHL (left)	=	ΣAAHL + ΣCHL		
		=	85 dB		
	NNIHD	=		13%	(Table A2: better ear 45, difference 40)
Difference:	NIHD	=		41% – 13%	
	Result	=		28%	

Example 10

Apportion the noise-induced hearing disability (NIHD) of 27% between the following five relevant episodes of noise exposure: episode 1 with employer A from 1952 to 1956 inclusive (5 years) at a daily noise exposure level ($L_{EP,d}$) of 98 dB(A) without hearing protection; episode 2 with employer B from 1957 to 1961 inclusive (5 years) at an $L_{EP,d}$ of 103 dB(A) without hearing protection; after a break of two years without noise exposure, episode 3 with employer C from 1964 to 1971 inclusive (8 years) at an $L_{EP,d}$ of 103 dB(A) without hearing protection; episode 4 with employer C from 1972 to 1979 inclusive (8 years) at an $L_{EP,d}$ of 103 dB(A) and understood to have worn the (unidentified) soft plastic earplugs then provided almost all the time exposed to noise; episode 5 with employer C from 1980 to 1987 inclusive (8 years) at an $L_{EP,d}$ of 103 dB(A) and understood to have consistently worn the (unidentified) earmuffs provided in 1980.

Method. Apply the procedure described in 10.1.2. For each episode of noise exposure calculate the product of the noise exposure duration in years (*T*) and $L_{EP,d}$, corrected for any use of hearing protection (see Appendix B), minus 84 dB(A). The NIHD is then apportioned in the ratio of these products.

Products:

Episode 1:	=	5 x (98 – 84)	=	70
Episode 2:	=	5 x (103 – 84)	=	95
Episode 3:	=	8 x (103 – 84)	=	152
Episode 4:	=	8 x [(103 – 10) – 84]	=	72
Episode 5:	=	8 x [(103 – 20) – 84]	=	0*
Total of 5 products			=	389

Relative proportions of the NIHD:

Episode 1:	=	70/389	=	0.18
Episode 2:	=	95/389	=	0.24
Episode 3:	=	152/389	=	0.39
Episode 4:	=	72/389	=	0.19
Episode 5:	=	0/389	=	0.00

Absolute NIHD values:

Episode 1:	=	0.18 x 27%	=	4.9%
Episode 2:	=	0.24 x 27%	=	6.6%
Episode 3:	=	0.39 x 27%	=	10.6%
Episode 4:	=	0.19 x 27%	=	5.0%
Episode 5:	=	0.00 x 27%	=	0.0%

Note: comparison between episodes 1 and 2 illustrates the effect of different noise levels. Comparison between episodes 2 and 3 illustrates the effect of different durations. Comparison between episodes 3, 4 and 5 illustrates the effect of no, insufficient and sufficient hearing protection.

*–8 counts as 0.

Appendix B
Guidelines on allowances to be made for the expected attenuation of noise by various types of hearing protector

In apportionment calculations (see 10.1.2), allowances have to be subtracted from the levels of noise at work during the years in which hearing protection was understood to have been properly used. Such allowances should only be made where it is believed that the hearing protection had been used for almost all the time that the individual was exposed to hazardous levels of noise.

If the particular protector used can be identified, its attenuation characteristics may be obtainable either from published data (e.g. Martin, 1977) or from information provided by its manufacturer. Account has then to be taken of the evidence that hearing protectors are less effective as worn in industry than as measured in the laboratory (Berger, 1983), their real-world attenuation being about 16 dB less for earplugs and 8 dB less for earmuffs.

Where the actual protector used cannot be identified with certainty, or its attenuation characteristics are not known, recourse may be necessary to the guidelines in Table B1. The table gives values for the mean real-world attenuation of A-weighted noise levels likely to be achieved for various classes of hearing protector.

Table B1 Expected real-world attenuation values for various classes of hearing protector.

Class of hearing protector	Attenuation (dB)
Dry cotton wool and music headphones	0
Waxed cotton wool	5
Soft plastic earplugs	10
Canal caps (suprameatal plugs on headband)	10
Personalized earmoulds	10
Glass down earplugs (e.g. Bilsom range)	15
Plastic foam earplugs (e.g. EAR range)	15
Earmuffs	20

These values may be used in apportionment calculations (see 10.1.2). They can also be used for diagnostic purposes (see 9.1.1), where the amount of hearing loss measured should quantitatively relate to the estimated noise exposures, the latter of course being adjusted for any use of hearing protection. However, they must *not* be used for general hearing conservation purposes where the aim is to select hearing protectors which give sufficient protection in a particular noise environment: for that purpose, the current Government regulations and associated noise guides (Health and Safety Executive, 1990) must be used.

Appendix C
Other considerations related to assessment

C1 Tinnitus

Previous British attempts (DHSS, 1973; Anon, 1983) to quantify hearing disability, particularly that associated with NIHL, have not included any description or mode of assessment of the tinnitus itself, nor any attempt to quantify any disability which may result from it. Certain settlement schemes consider that tinnitus may be assessed as mild, moderate or severe, but the assessment of the severity of the symptom itself, and its effects on the person and the prognosis is left to the medical examiner. In these circumstances, each individual examiner would devise his own method based on his clinical practice and experience, but a descriptive scale such as 'Trivial – Slight – Moderate – Severe – Very Severe' is helpful. 'Severity' of tinnitus depends not only on the characteristics of the tinnitus *per se*, but also on the effects of the tinnitus on the individual.

Attempts have been made by several workers in different centres to assess the pitch, bandwidth, loudness, and maskability of the tinnitus. Matching and masking techniques frequently lead to spurious results and this is particularly the case where sounds are multiple or bizarre. Synthesizers have been employed also but specialized equipment for tinnitus matching is not widely available nor likely to be very satisfactory. In any event, the results are difficult to interpret in terms of severity, which depends in the individual case on many other factors, most of them unmeasurable (Hinchcliffe and King, 1992).

Leading questions should be avoided wherever possible. Case notes and medicolegal reports should indicate what questions were asked, their order, the answers and any information volunteered. Although tinnitus can be regarded as a likely concomitant in about 50% of cases of NIHL, as with all types of hearing loss, it is considered inappropriate to attempt quantification of these symptoms in terms of additional disability. It should be left to the judgement of the medical examiner to comment on the claimant's reaction to tinnitus, should he suffer from it or whether it be part of his claim. The assessment has to be related to the claimant's description, but paying due regard to any descriptive or audiometric inconsistencies, and to the claimant's motivation.

Apportionment of tinnitus between episodes of noise exposure is not a simple matter. If there is no evidence to the contrary, any apportionment should be proportional to the noise-induced hearing disability. In other cases, it should be left to the judgement of the medical examiner. This matter has been discussed by Hinchcliffe and King (1992).

C2 *Noise-induced vestibular malfunction*

Although noise levels over about 90 dB(A) can cause vertigo or imbalance in some cases of inner-ear disorder, and noise levels over about 130 dB (dB(A) or dB peak) can sometimes do so in persons with normal ears, these so-called 'Tullio effects' are not sustained after the noise exposure has ceased. While there have been reports claiming that noise exposure can cause permanent damage to the vestibular system, a recent review of the literature (Hinchcliffe, Coles and King, 1992) failed to provide convincing evidence for this.

C3 *Use of hearing aids*

When assessing hearing disability for compensation settlement schemes that are applied to large numbers of claimants, this should be calculated according to the unaided state. This is partly due to the relatively small reduction of disability achieved by hearing aids in most compensable forms of hearing disorder, and also because of the multitude of audiological, economic, social and administrative variables involved in predicting, obtaining and assessing benefit from hearing aid(s).

In common-law cases where each case is considered on its own merits, however, these variables will have to be considered individually for each claimant. Relief in this context is a combination of reduction of disability, offset by such factors as the cost, inconvenience and perhaps discomfort involved. With respect to use of hearing aids in cases of sensorineural hearing loss, it should be recognized that they are usually less effective, less easy to use and more uncomfortable than, for example, spectacles when the latter are used for correction of the most common (refraction) errors of vision.

In all cases, an assessment should be accompanied by statements concerning any special provision that needs to be made for the individual. Often this will entail prescription of suitable hearing aids and other devices intended to mitigate the effects of the disability (e.g. TV amplifier, Teletext adaptor, extra-loud telephone ringer). Not all such apparatus will be available from public funds. Furthermore, public provision may not match the performance obtainable with commercially available instruments. For example, binaural hearing aids are known to give greater benefit than the monaural systems generally provided by National Health Service (NHS) departments, whilst some hearing-impaired people report greater benefit from in-the-ear hearing aids than from the behind-the-ear instruments routinely provided by the NHS. The medical examiner should give details of all such apparatus that might be expected to help the claimant, and its costs if not generally available from public funds. Such costs should include the purchase price, running costs and estimates of the cost of repairs and replacements.

References

AAOO (1959). Guide for the evaluation of hearing impairment (Report of the Subcommittee on Noise of the Committee on Conservation of Hearing). *Transactions of the American Academy of Ophthalmology and Otolaryngology* **63**, 236–238.

Alberti, P.W. (1987). Noise and the ear. In *Scott–Brown's Otolaryngology*, Volume 2, *Adult Audiology* (ed.D. Stephens). Guildford: Butterworths, 594–641.

Alberti, P. W., Morgan, P. P. and Czuba, I. (1978). Speech and pure-tone audiometry as a screen for exaggerated hearing loss in industrial claims. *Acta Oto-Laryngologica* **87**, 728–731.

Anon (1981). Recommended procedure for pure tone audiometry using a manually operated instrument. *British Journal of Audiology* **15**, 213–216.

Anon (1983). BAOL/BSA method for assessment of hearing disability. *British Journal of Audiology* **17**, 203–212.

Atherley, G.R.C. and Noble, W.G. (1971). Clinical picture of occupational hearing loss obtained with the Hearing Measurement Scale. In *Occupational Hearing Loss* (ed. D.W. Robinson). London: Academic Press, 193–206.

Berger, C.H. (1983). Using the NRR to estimate the real world performance of hearing protectors. *Sound and Vibration* **17**, 12–18.

BS 2497 Specification for a reference zero for the calibration of pure-tone audiometers Part 4:1972 Normal threshold of hearing for pure tones by bone conduction. London: British Standards Institution (withdrawn).

BS 2497 Standard reference zero for the calibration of pure tone air conduction audiometers Part 5:1988 Standard reference zero using an acoustic coupler complying with BS 4668. London: British Standards Institution.

BS 2497 Standard reference zero for the calibration of pure tone air conduction audiometers Part 6:1988 Standard reference zero using an artificial ear complying with BS 4669. London: British Standards Institution.

BS 2475:1964 Octave and one-third octave band-pass filters. London: British Standards Institution.

BS 4009:1975 An artificial mastoid for the calibration of bone vibrators used in hearing aids and audiometers. London: British Standards Institution (withdrawn).

BS 4009:1991 Specification for artificial mastoids for the calibration of bone vibrators used in hearing aids and audiometers. London: British Standards Institution.

BS 4668:1971 Specification for an acoustic coupler (IEC reference type) for the calibration of earphones used in audiometry. London: British Standards Institution.

BS 4669:1971 Specification for an artificial ear of the wide band type for the calibration of earphones used in audiometry. London: British Standards Institution.

BS 5966:1980 Specification for audiometers. London: British Standards Institution.

BS 5969:1981 Specification for sound level meters. London: British Standards Institution.

BS 6655:1986 Pure tone air conduction threshold audiometry for hearing conservation purposes. London: British Standards Institution.

BS 6698:1986 Specification for integrating-averaging sound level meters. London: British Standards Institution.

BS 6950:1988 Standard reference zero for the calibration of pure tone bone conduction audiometers. London: British Standards Institution.

BS 6951:1988 Threshold of hearing by air conduction as a function of age and sex for otologically normal persons. London: British Standards Institution.

BS 7113:1989 Specification for reference levels for narrow-band masking noise. London: British Standards Institution.

BS 7189:1989 Specification for sound calibrators. London: British Standards Institution.

BSA (1985). Recommended procedures for pure-tone bone-conduction audiometry without masking using a manually operated instrument. *British Journal of Audiology* **19**, 281–282.

BSA (1986). Recommendations for masking in pure tone audiometry. *British Journal of Audiology* **20**, 307–314.

BSA (1989). British Society of Audiology – recommended format for audiogram forms. *British Journal of Audiology* **23**, 265–266.

Bunch, C.C., Fowler, E.P. and Sabine, P.E. (1942). Tentative standard procedure for evaluating the percentage of useful hearing loss in medico-legal cases. *Journal of the American Medical Association* **119**, 1108–1109.

CHABA (1975). Compensation formula for hearing loss. NAS-NRC Committee on Hearing, Bioacoustics and Biomechanics, Report of Working Group 77, Washington DC.

Coles, R.R.A. (1967). External meatus closure by audiometer earphone. *Journal of Speech and Hearing Disorders* **32**, 296–297.

Coles, R.R.A. (1975). Relationships between noise-induced threshold shifts, morphological change and social handicap. *Symposia of the Zoological Society of London* No. 37, 107–120.

Coles, R. R. A. (1982). Non-organic hearing loss. In *Butterworths International Medical Reviews, Otolaryngology 1, Otology* (eds A.G. Gibb and M.C.W. Smith). London: Butterworths, 150–176.

Coles, R.R.A., Lutman, M.E. and Robinson, D.W. (1991). The limited accuracy of bone-conduction audiometry: its significance in medicolegal assessments. *Journal of Laryngology and Otology* **105**, 518–521.

Coles, R. R. A. and Mason, S. M. (1984). The results of cortical electric response audiometry in medico-legal investigations. *British Journal of Audiology* **18**, 71–78.

Coles, R. R. A. and Priede, V. M. (1971). Non-organic overlay in noise-induced hearing loss. *Proceedings of the Royal Society of Medicine* **64**, 194–199.

Coles, R. R. A. and Priede, V. M. (1976). Speech discrimination tests in investigation of sensorineural hearing loss. *Journal of Laryngology and Otology* **90**, 1081–1092.

Davis, A.C. (1989). The prevalence of hearing impairment and reported hearing disability among adults in Great Britain. *International Journal of Epidemiology* **18**, 911–917.

Davis, H. (1971). A historical introduction. In *Occupational Hearing Loss* (ed. D.W. Robinson). London and New York: Academic Press, 7–12.

Department of Health and Social Security (1973). National Insurance (Industrial Injuries) Act 1965: Occupational deafness. Cmnd 5461. London: HMSO.

Fletcher, H. (1929). *Speech and Hearing*. London: Macmillan, Chap.VI.

Fletcher, H. (1953). *Speech and Hearing in Communication*. Princeton, NJ: van Nostrand, Chap.20.

Fournier, J. E. (1956). La dépistage de la simulation auditive. In *Exposés Annuels d'Oto-Rhino-Laryngologie*, pp. 107–126. Paris: Masson et Cie. (Also translation No. 8 (1958) of the Beltone Institute for Hearing Research, Chicago: *The detection of auditory malingering.)*

Fowler, E. P. (1942). A simple method of measuring percentage of capacity for hearing speech. *Archives of Otolaryngology* 36, 874–890.

Ginnold, R.E. (1979). Occupational hearing loss: Workers' compensation under State and Federal programs. Report EPA-550/9-79-101. Washington DC: US Environmental Protection Agency.

Habib, R.G. and Hinchcliffe, R. (1978). Subjective magnitude of auditory impairment: a pilot study. *Audiology* **17**, 68–76.

Hardick, E.J., Melnick, W., Hawes, N.A., Pillian, J.P., Stephens, R.G. and Perlmutter, D.J. (1980). Compensation for hearing loss for employees under jurisdiction of the US Department of Labor: benefit formula and assessment procedures. Contract report J-9-E-9-0205. Columbus, OH: Ohio State University.

Harris, D. A. (1958). Rapid and simple technique for detection of non-organic hearing loss. *Archives of Otolaryngology* **68**, 758–760.

Health and Safety Executive (1989). Noise at work. Noise guide no. 1. Legal duties of employers to prevent damage to hearing. London: HMSO.

Health and Safety Executive (1990). Noise at work. Noise guide no. 5. Type and selection of personal ear protectors. London: HMSO.

Hinchcliffe, R. (1992). Sound, infrasound and ultrasound. In *Hunter's Diseases of Occupations* (eds A. Raffle, P. Adams, P. Baxter, P. and W. R. Lee). London: Hodder and Stoughton.

Hinchcliffe, R. and King, P. F. (1992) Medicolegal aspects of tinnitus. I: Medicolegal position and current state of knowledge. *Journal of Audiological Medicine* in press.

Hinchcliffe, R. Coles, R. R. A. and King, P. F. (1992) Occupational noise-induced vestibular malfunction? *British Journal of Industrial Medicine* 49, 63–65.

IEC 373:1990 Mechanical coupler for measurements on bone vibrators, 2nd edition. Geneva: International Electrotechnical Commission.

IEC 645-2 (at the draft stage) Equipment for speech audiometry. Geneva: International Electrotechnical Commission.

IEC 1027:1991 Instruments for the measurement of aural acoustic impedance/admittance. Geneva: International Electrotechnical Commission.

ISO 389:1991 Acoustics – standard reference zero for the calibration of pure-tone audiometers, 3rd edn. Geneva: International Organization for Standardization.

ISO 7029:1984 Acoustics – threshold of hearing by air conduction as a function of age and sex for otologically normal persons. Geneva: International Organization for Standardization.

ISO 8253-1:1989 Acoustics – Audiometric test methods – Part 1: Basic pure tone air and bone conduction threshold audiometry. Geneva: International Organization for Standardization.

Kell, R.L., Pearson, J.C.G., Acton, W.I. and Taylor, W. (1971). Social effects of hearing loss due to weaving noise. In *Occupational Hearing Loss* (ed. D.W. Robinson) London: Academic Press.

Kerr, A. G., Gillespie, W. J. and Easton, J. M. (1975). Deafness: a simple test for malingering. *British Journal of Audiology* **9**, 24–26.

Lutman, M. E. (1992). Apportionment of noise-indicated hearing disability and its prognosis in a medicolegal context. A modelling study. *British Journal of Audiology* in press.

Lutman, M. E. and Robinson, D. W. (1992). Quantification of hearing disability for medicolegal purposes based on self-rating. *British Journal of Audiology* in press.

Lutman, M.E., Brown, E.J. and Coles, R.R.A. (1987). Self-reported disability and handicap in the population in relation to pure-tone threshold, age, sex and type of hearing loss. *British Journal of Audiology* **21**, 45–58.

Macrae, J.H. and Brigden, D.N. (1973). Auditory threshold impairment and everyday speech reception. *Audiology* **12**, 272–290.

MacKeith, N.W. and Coles, R.R.A. (1971). Binaural advantage in hearing of speech. *Journal of Laryngology and Otology* **85**, 213–232.

Martin, A.M. (1977). The acoustic attenuation characteristics of 26 hearing protectors evaluated following the British Standard procedure. *Annals of Occupational Hygiene* **20**, 229–246.

Merluzzi, F. and Hinchcliffe, R. (1973). Threshold of subjective auditory handicap. *Audiology* **12**, 65–69.

Noble, W.G. (1978). *Assessment of Impaired Hearing*. New York: Academic Press.

Robinson, D.W. (1985). The audiogram in hearing loss due to noise: a probability test to uncover other causation. *Annals of Occupational Hygiene* **29**, 477–493.

Robinson, D.W. (1987). Noise exposure and hearing: a new look at the experimental data. Health and Safety Executive Contract Report No. 1/1987. Bootle: HSE Sales Point.

Robinson, D.W. (1988a). Tables for the estimation of hearing impairment due to noise for otologically normal persons and for a typical unscreened population, as a function of age and duration of exposure. Health and Safety Executive Contract Report No. 2/1988. Bootle: HSE Sales Point.

Robinson, D.W. (1988b). Threshold of hearing as a function of age and sex for the typical unscreened population. *British Journal of Audiology* **22**, 5–20.

Robinson, D.W. (1991a). Long-term repeatability of the pure-tone hearing threshold and its relation to noise exposure. *British Journal of Audiology* **25**, 219–236.

Robinson, D.W. (1991b). Relation between hearing threshold level and its component parts. *British Journal of Audiology* **25**, 93–103.

Robinson, D.W. (1992). Background noise in rooms used for pure-tone audiometry in disability assessment. *British Journal of Audiology* in press.

Robinson, D.W. and Shipton, M.S. (1977). Tables for the estimation of noise-induced hearing loss. Report Ac 61, 2nd edition. Teddington: National Physical Laboratory.

Robinson, D.W. and Sutton, G.J. (1978). A comparative analysis of data on the relation of pure-tone audiometric thresholds to age. NPL Acoustics Report Ac 84. Teddington, National Physical Laboratory.

Robinson, D.W. and Sutton, G.J. (1979). Age effect in hearing – a comparative analysis of published threshold data. *Audiology* **18**, 320–334.

Robinson, D.W., Wilkins, P.A., Thyer, N.J. and Lawes, J.F. (1984). Auditory impairment and the onset of disability and handicap in noise-induced hearing loss. ISVR Technical Report No.126, University of Southampton.

Robinson, P.C. (1978). Fundamental issues in the audiological assessment of compensation claimants. In *Occupational Hearing Loss Conservation and Compensation* (eds R.L. Waugh and J.H. Macrae). Proceedings of the 1978 conference of the Australian Acoustical Society, 209–224.

Sabine, P.E. (1942). On estimating the percentage loss of useful hearing. *Transactions of the American Academy of Ophthalmology and Otolaryngology* **46**, 179–196.

Shipton, M.S. (1979). Tables relating pure-tone audiometric threshold to age. NPL Acoustics Report Ac 94. Teddington: National Physical Laboratory.

Shipton, M.S. (1987). Recommendations for organising the calibration of pure-tone audiometers. NPL Acoustics Report Ac 112. Teddington: National Physical Laboratory.

Stephens, S.D.G. (1981). Clinical audiometry. In *Audiology and Audiological Medicine*, Vol.1 (ed. H.A.Beagley). Oxford: Oxford University Press, 365–370.

Suter, A.H. (1978). The ability of mildly hearing-impaired individuals to discriminate speech in noise. Report EPA–550/9–78–100. Washington DC: US Environmental Protection Agency.

Tyler, R.S. and Smith, P.A. (1983). Sentence identification in noise and hearing-handicap questionnaires. *Scandinavian Audiology* **12**, 285–292.

Webster, J.C. (1964). Important frequencies in noise-masked speech. *Archives of Otolaryngology* **80**, 494–504.

Annex A
Tables for use in calculating disability and apportionment

Table A1	Median age-associated hearing threshold levels for males and females
Table A2	Percentage disability as a function of better-ear HTL and asymmetry
Table A3	Percentage disability as a function of age for males and females, calculated using Tables A1 and A2
Table A4	Products of excess noise level above 84 dB(A) times exposure duration (used for apportionment calculation)

Table A1 **Median age associated hearing threshold levels for males and females. Values are based on ISO 7029 and are summed over the frequencies 1, 2 and 3 kHz (ΣAAHL), and extrapolated to include ages up to 80 years (italics). Values are given to the nearest 5 dB.**

ΣAAHL (dB)			ΣAAHL (dB)			ΣAAHL (dB)		
Age	M	F	Age	M	F	Age	M	F
18	0	0	39	10	10	60	40	30
19	0	0	40	10	10	61	40	30
20	0	0	41	10	10	62	45	35
21	0	0	42	15	10	63	45	35
22	0	0	43	15	10	64	50	35
23	0	0	44	15	10	65	50	40
24	0	0	45	15	15	66	50	40
25	0	0	46	20	15	67	55	40
26	0	0	47	20	15	68	55	45
27	0	0	48	20	15	69	60	45
28	0	0	49	20	15	70	60	45
29	5	0	50	25	20	*71*	*65*	*50*
30	5	0	51	25	20	*72*	*65*	*50*
31	5	5	52	25	20	*73*	*70*	*55*
32	5	5	53	30	20	*74*	*70*	*55*
33	5	5	54	30	25	*75*	*75*	*55*
34	5	5	55	30	25	*76*	*75*	*60*
35	5	5	56	30	25	*77*	*80*	*60*
36	5	5	57	35	25	*78*	*80*	*65*
37	10	5	58	35	30	*79*	*85*	*65*
38	10	5	59	35	30	*80*	*85*	*65*

Table A2 Percentage disability as a function of better-ear HTL and asymmetry. Rows correspond to HTLs in the better ear summed over 1, 2 and 3 kHz (ΣH). Columns correspond to differences in HTLs of better and worse ears, summed over the frequencies 1, 2 and 3 kHz.

ΣH	Difference in HTLs of better and worse ears (summed over 1, 2 and 3 kHz)																													
	0	5	10	15	20	25	30	35	40	45	50	55	60	65	70	75	80	85	90	95	100	105	110	115	120	125	130	135	140	145	150
-30	0	0	0	0	1	1	2	2	3	3	4	4	4	5	5	6	6	6	7	7	7	8	8	9	9	9	10	10	10	11	11
-25	0	0	1	1	1	2	2	3	3	3	4	4	5	5	6	6	6	7	7	7	8	8	9	9	9	10	10	10	11	11	11
-20	1	1	1	1	2	2	3	3	3	4	4	5	5	6	6	6	7	7	8	8	8	9	9	9	10	10	10	11	11	12	12
-15	1	1	1	2	2	3	3	3	4	4	5	5	6	6	7	7	7	8	8	8	9	9	10	10	10	11	11	11	12	12	12
-10	1	2	2	2	2	3	3	4	4	5	5	6	6	7	7	7	8	8	9	9	9	10	10	10	11	11	12	12	12	13	13
-5	2	2	2	2	3	3	4	4	5	5	6	6	7	7	8	8	8	9	9	10	10	10	11	11	11	12	12	12	13	13	13
0	2	2	3	3	3	4	5	5	6	6	6	7	7	8	8	9	9	9	10	10	11	11	11	12	12	12	13	13	13	14	14
5	3	3	3	3	4	5	5	6	6	7	7	8	8	8	9	9	10	10	10	11	11	12	12	12	13	13	13	14	14	14	15
10	3	4	4	4	5	5	6	6	7	7	8	8	9	9	10	10	10	11	11	12	12	12	13	13	13	14	14	14	15	15	15
15	4	4	4	5	5	6	6	7	7	8	8	9	9	10	10	11	11	12	12	12	13	13	13	14	14	15	15	15	16	16	16
20	4	5	5	5	6	7	7	8	8	9	9	10	10	11	11	12	12	12	13	13	14	14	14	15	15	15	16	16	16	17	17
25	5	5	6	6	7	7	8	8	9	9	10	11	11	11	12	12	13	13	14	14	14	15	15	15	16	16	17	17	17	18	18
30	6	6	7	7	7	8	9	9	10	10	11	11	12	12	13	13	14	14	14	15	15	16	16	16	17	17	17	18	18	18	19
35	7	7	7	8	8	9	10	10	11	11	12	12	13	13	14	14	15	15	15	16	16	17	17	17	18	18	18	19	19	19	20
40	7	8	8	9	9	10	10	11	12	12	13	13	14	14	15	15	16	16	16	17	17	18	18	18	19	19	19	20	20	20	21
45	8	9	9	9	10	11	11	12	13	13	14	14	15	15	16	16	17	17	17	18	18	19	19	19	20	20	20	21	21	21	22
50	9	10	10	10	11	12	12	13	14	14	15	15	16	16	17	17	18	18	19	19	19	20	20	20	21	21	22	22	22	22	23
55	10	10	11	11	12	13	13	14	15	15	16	16	17	17	18	18	19	19	20	20	21	21	21	22	22	22	23	23	23	24	24

Table A2 continued

ΣH	Difference in HTLs of better and worse ears (summed over 1, 2 and 3 kHz)																													
	0	5	10	15	20	25	30	35	40	45	50	55	60	65	70	75	80	85	90	95	100	105	110	115	120	125	130	135	140	145	150
60	11	12	12	12	13	14	15	15	16	16	17	18	18	19	19	20	20	20	21	21	22	22	22	23	23	24	24	24	24	25	25
65	12	13	13	14	14	15	16	16	17	18	18	19	19	20	20	21	21	22	22	23	23	23	24	24	24	25	25	25	26	26	26
70	13	14	14	15	16	16	17	18	18	19	20	20	21	21	22	22	23	23	23	24	24	25	25	25	26	26	26	27	27	27	28
75	14	15	15	16	17	18	18	19	20	20	21	21	22	22	23	23	24	24	25	25	26	26	26	27	27	27	28	28	28	29	29
80	16	16	17	17	18	19	20	20	21	22	22	23	23	24	24	25	25	26	26	27	27	27	28	28	28	29	29	29	30	30	30
85	17	17	18	19	19	20	21	22	22	23	24	24	25	25	26	26	27	27	28	28	28	29	29	30	30	30	31	31	31	32	32
90	18	19	19	20	21	22	22	23	24	24	25	26	26	27	27	28	28	29	29	30	30	30	31	31	31	32	32	32	33	33	33
95	19	20	21	21	22	23	24	25	25	26	27	27	28	28	29	29	30	30	31	31	32	32	32	33	33	33	34	34	34	35	35
100	21	22	22	23	24	25	25	26	27	28	28	29	29	30	30	31	31	32	32	33	33	34	34	34	35	35	35	36	36	36	36
105	22	23	24	24	25	26	27	28	29	29	30	30	31	32	32	33	33	34	34	34	35	35	36	36	36	37	37	37	37	38	38
110	24	25	25	26	27	28	29	29	30	31	32	32	33	33	34	34	35	35	36	36	36	37	37	38	38	38	39	39	39	39	40
115	25	26	27	28	29	30	30	31	32	33	33	34	34	35	36	36	37	37	37	38	38	39	39	39	40	40	40	41	41	41	41
120	27	28	29	29	30	31	32	33	34	34	35	36	36	37	37	38	38	39	39	40	40	40	41	41	41	42	42	42	43	43	43
125	29	30	30	31	32	33	34	35	35	36	37	37	38	39	39	40	40	41	41	41	42	42	42	43	43	43	44	44	44	45	45
130	31	31	32	33	34	35	36	37	37	38	39	39	40	40	41	42	42	42	43	43	44	44	44	45	45	45	46	46	46	46	47
135	32	33	34	35	36	37	38	38	39	40	41	41	42	42	43	43	44	44	45	45	45	46	46	46	47	47	47	48	48	48	48
140	34	35	36	37	38	39	40	40	41	42	42	43	44	44	45	45	46	46	47	47	47	48	48	48	49	49	49	49	50	50	50
145	36	37	38	39	40	41	41	42	43	44	44	45	46	46	47	47	48	48	48	49	49	50	50	50	51	51	51	51	52	52	52
150	38	39	40	41	42	43	43	44	45	46	46	47	48	48	49	49	50	50	50	51	51	51	52	52	52	53	53	53	53	54	54

Table A2 continued

ΣH	Difference in HTLs of better and worse ears (summed over 1, 2 and 3 kHz)																													
	0	5	10	15	20	25	30	35	40	45	50	55	60	65	70	75	80	85	90	95	100	105	110	115	120	125	130	135	140	145	150
155	40	41	42	43	44	44	45	46	47	48	48	49	50	50	51	51	52	52	52	53	53	53	54	54	54	55	55	55	55	55	56
160	42	43	44	45	46	46	47	48	49	50	50	51	51	52	53	53	53	54	54	55	55	55	56	56	56	56	57	57	57	57	58
165	44	45	46	47	48	48	49	50	51	52	52	53	53	54	54	55	55	56	56	56	57	57	57	58	58	58	58	59	59	59	59
170	46	47	48	49	50	50	51	52	53	54	54	55	55	56	56	57	57	58	58	58	59	59	59	60	60	60	60	61	61	61	61
175	48	49	50	51	52	52	53	54	55	56	56	57	57	58	58	59	59	60	60	60	61	61	61	61	62	62	62	62	63	63	63
180	50	51	52	53	54	54	55	56	57	57	58	59	59	60	60	61	61	61	62	62	62	63	63	63	63	64	64	64	64	65	65
185	52	53	54	55	56	56	57	58	59	59	60	61	61	62	62	62	63	63	64	64	64	64	65	65	65	65	66	66	66	66	66
190	54	55	56	57	58	58	59	60	61	61	62	62	63	63	64	64	65	65	65	66	66	66	67	67	67	67	67	68	68	68	68
195	56	57	58	59	59	60	61	62	63	63	64	64	65	65	66	66	66	67	67	67	68	68	68	68	69	69	69	69	69	70	70
200	58	59	60	61	61	62	63	64	64	65	66	66	67	67	67	68	68	69	69	69	69	70	70	70	70	71	71	71	71	71	71
205	60	61	62	62	63	64	65	66	66	67	67	68	68	69	69	70	70	70	71	71	71	71	72	72	72	72	72	73	73	73	73
210	62	63	63	64	65	66	67	67	68	69	69	70	70	71	71	71	72	72	72	72	73	73	73	73	74	74	74	74	74	74	75
215	64	65	65	66	67	68	68	69	70	70	71	71	72	72	73	73	73	74	74	74	74	74	75	75	75	75	75	76	76	76	
220	65	66	67	68	69	70	70	71	71	72	72	73	73	74	74	74	75	75	75	76	76	76	76	76	77	77	77	77	77		
225	67	68	69	70	70	71	72	72	73	74	74	75	75	75	76	76	76	77	77	77	77	77	78	78	78	78	78	78			
230	69	70	71	71	72	73	73	74	75	75	76	76	76	77	77	77	78	78	78	78	79	79	79	79	79	80	80				
235	71	72	72	73	74	74	75	76	76	77	77	78	78	78	79	79	79	79	80	80	80	80	80	81	81	81					
240	72	73	74	75	75	76	77	77	78	78	79	79	79	80	80	80	80	81	81	81	81	81	82	82	82						
245	74	75	76	76	77	77	78	79	79	79	80	80	81	81	81	81	82	82	82	82	83	83	83	83							

Table A2 continued

ΣH	Difference in HTLs of better and worse ears (summed over 1, 2 and 3 kHz)																													
	0	5	10	15	20	25	30	35	40	45	50	55	60	65	70	75	80	85	90	95	100	105	110	115	120	125	130	135	140	145	150
250	76	76	77	78	78	79	79	80	80	81	81	82	82	82	82	83	83	83	83	84	84	84	84								
255	77	78	78	79	80	80	81	81	82	82	82	83	83	83	84	84	84	84	84	85	85	85									
260	79	79	80	80	81	82	82	83	83	83	84	84	84	85	85	85	85	85	86	86	86										
265	80	81	81	82	82	83	83	84	84	84	85	85	85	86	86	86	86	86	87	87											
270	81	82	82	83	83	84	84	85	85	86	86	86	86	87	87	87	87	87	88												
275	83	83	84	84	85	85	86	86	86	87	87	87	87	88	88	88	88	88													
280	84	84	85	85	86	86	87	87	87	88	88	88	88	89	89	89	89														
285	85	85	86	86	87	87	88	88	88	88	89	89	89	89	90	90															
290	86	86	87	87	88	88	88	89	89	89	90	90	90	90	90																
295	87	87	88	88	89	89	89	90	90	90	90	91	91	91																	
300	88	88	89	89	90	90	90	90	91	91	91	91	92																		
305	89	89	90	90	90	91	91	91	91	92	92	92																			
310	90	90	90	91	91	91	92	92	92	92	93																				
315	90	91	91	91	92	92	92	93	93	93																					
320	91	92	92	92	92	93	93	93	93																						
325	92	92	93	93	93	93	94	94																							
330	93	93	93	93	94	94	94																								
335	93	93	94	94	94	94																									
340	94	94	94	94	95																										

Table A2 continued

ΣH	Difference in HTLs of better and worse ears (summed over 1, 2 and 3 kHz)																														
	0	5	10	15	20	25	30	35	40	45	50	55	60	65	70	75	80	85	90	95	100	105	110	115	120	125	130	135	140	145	150
345	94	95	95	95																											
350	95	95	95																												
355	95	95																													
360	96																														

Table A3 **Percentage disability as a function of age for males and females, calculated using Tables A1 and A2. Values applicable if the only cause of hearing impairment is age-associated hearing loss (AAHL). Values in italics are based on extrapolation beyond the scope of ISO 7029 (see Table A1).**

Disability (%)			Disability (%)			Disability (%)		
Age	M	F	Age	M	F	Age	M	F
18	2	2	39	3	3	60	7	6
19	2	2	40	3	3	61	7	6
20	2	2	41	3	3	62	8	7
21	2	2	42	4	3	63	8	7
22	2	2	43	4	3	64	9	7
23	2	2	44	4	3	65	9	7
24	2	2	45	4	4	66	9	7
25	2	2	46	4	4	67	10	7
26	2	2	47	4	4	68	10	8
27	2	2	48	4	4	69	11	8
28	2	2	49	4	4	70	11	8
29	3	2	50	5	4	*71*	*12*	*9*
30	3	2	51	5	4	*72*	*12*	*9*
31	3	3	52	5	4	*73*	*13*	*10*
32	3	3	53	6	4	*74*	*13*	*10*
33	3	3	54	6	5	*75*	*14*	*10*
34	3	3	55	6	5	*76*	*14*	*11*
35	3	3	56	6	5	*77*	*16*	*11*
36	3	3	57	7	5	*78*	*16*	*12*
37	3	3	58	7	6	*79*	*17*	*12*
38	3	3	59	7	6	*80*	*17*	*12*

Table A4. **Products of excess noise level above 84 dB(A) times exposure duration. Columns correspond to actual noise levels expressed as equivalent continuous sound pressure levels ($L_{EP,d}$). Rows correspond to duration (T) in years.**

T	Equivalent continuous sound level ($L_{EP,d}$) in dB(A)																				
years	85	86	87	88	89	90	91	92	93	94	95	96	97	98	99	100	101	102	103	104	105
1	1	2	3	4	5	6	7	8	9	10	11	12	13	14	15	16	17	18	19	20	21
2	2	4	6	8	10	12	14	16	18	20	22	24	26	28	30	32	34	36	38	40	42
3	3	6	9	12	15	18	21	24	27	30	33	36	39	42	45	48	51	54	57	60	63
4	4	8	12	16	20	24	28	32	36	40	44	48	52	56	60	64	68	72	76	80	84
5	5	10	15	20	25	30	35	40	45	50	55	60	65	70	75	80	85	90	95	100	105
6	6	12	18	24	30	36	42	48	54	60	66	72	78	84	90	96	102	108	114	120	126
7	7	14	21	28	35	42	49	56	63	70	77	84	91	98	105	112	119	126	133	140	147
8	8	16	24	32	40	48	56	64	72	80	88	96	104	112	120	128	136	144	152	160	168
9	9	18	27	36	45	54	63	72	81	90	99	108	117	126	135	144	153	162	171	180	189
10	10	20	30	40	50	60	70	80	90	100	110	120	130	140	150	160	170	180	190	200	210
11	11	22	33	44	55	66	77	88	99	110	121	132	143	154	165	176	187	198	209	220	231
12	12	24	36	48	60	72	84	96	108	120	132	144	156	168	180	192	204	216	228	240	252
13	13	26	39	52	65	78	91	104	117	130	143	156	169	182	195	208	221	234	247	260	273
14	14	28	42	56	70	84	98	112	126	140	154	168	182	196	210	224	238	252	266	280	294
15	15	30	45	60	75	90	105	120	135	150	165	180	195	210	225	240	255	270	285	300	315
16	16	32	48	64	80	96	112	128	144	160	176	192	208	224	240	256	272	288	304	320	336
17	17	34	51	68	85	102	119	136	153	170	187	204	221	238	255	272	289	306	323	340	357
18	18	36	54	72	90	108	126	144	162	180	198	216	234	252	270	288	306	324	342	360	378

Table A4 continued

T years	Equivalent continuous sound level ($L_{EP,d}$) in dB(A)																				
	85	86	87	88	89	90	91	92	93	94	95	96	97	98	99	100	101	102	103	104	105
19	19	38	57	76	95	114	133	152	171	190	209	228	247	266	285	304	323	342	361	380	399
20	20	40	60	80	100	120	140	160	180	200	220	240	260	280	300	320	340	360	380	400	420
21	21	42	63	84	105	126	147	168	189	210	231	252	273	294	315	336	357	378	399	420	441
22	22	44	66	88	110	132	154	176	198	220	242	264	286	308	330	352	374	396	418	440	462
23	23	46	69	92	115	138	161	184	207	230	253	276	299	322	345	368	391	414	437	460	483
24	24	48	72	96	120	144	168	192	216	240	264	288	312	336	360	384	408	432	456	480	504
25	25	50	75	100	125	150	175	200	225	250	275	300	325	350	375	400	425	450	475	500	525
26	26	52	78	104	130	156	182	208	234	260	286	312	338	364	390	416	442	468	494	520	546
27	27	54	81	108	135	162	189	216	243	270	297	324	351	378	405	432	459	486	513	540	567
28	28	56	84	112	140	168	196	224	252	280	308	336	364	392	420	448	476	504	532	560	588
29	29	58	87	116	145	174	203	232	261	290	319	348	377	406	435	464	493	522	551	580	609
30	30	60	90	120	150	180	210	240	270	300	330	360	390	420	450	480	510	540	570	600	630
31	31	62	93	124	155	186	217	248	279	310	341	372	403	434	465	496	527	558	589	620	651
32	32	64	96	128	160	192	224	256	288	320	352	384	416	448	480	512	544	576	608	640	672
33	33	66	99	132	165	198	231	264	297	330	363	396	429	462	495	528	561	594	627	660	693
34	34	68	102	136	170	204	238	272	306	340	374	408	442	476	510	544	578	612	646	680	714
35	35	70	105	140	175	210	245	280	315	350	385	420	455	490	525	560	595	630	665	700	735
36	36	72	108	144	180	216	252	288	324	360	396	432	468	504	540	576	612	648	684	720	756
37	37	74	111	148	185	222	259	296	333	370	407	444	481	518	555	592	629	666	703	740	777

Table A4 continued

T	Equivalent continuous sound level ($L_{EP,d}$) in dB(A)																				
years	85	86	87	88	89	90	91	92	93	94	95	96	97	98	99	100	101	102	103	104	105
38	38	76	114	152	190	228	266	304	342	380	418	456	494	532	570	608	646	684	722	760	798
39	39	78	117	156	195	234	273	312	351	390	429	468	507	546	585	624	663	702	741	780	819
40	40	80	120	160	200	240	280	320	360	400	440	480	520	560	600	640	680	720	760	800	840
41	41	82	123	164	205	246	287	328	369	410	451	492	533	574	615	656	697	738	779	820	861
42	42	84	126	168	210	252	294	336	378	420	462	504	546	588	630	672	714	756	798	840	882
43	43	86	129	172	215	258	301	344	387	430	473	516	559	602	645	688	731	774	817	860	903
44	44	88	132	176	220	264	308	352	396	440	484	528	572	616	660	704	748	792	836	880	924
45	45	90	135	180	225	270	315	360	405	450	495	540	585	630	675	720	765	810	855	900	945